EXCELLENCE IN HEALTH CARE MANAGEMENT

Edited by

ALISON MORTON-COOPER, *MEd, RGN*
and
MARGARET BAMFORD, *PhD, MSc, RGN, DASTE, OHNC, DN Cert, Teaching Cert*

Blackwell
Science

Copyright © 1997 by Alison Morton-Cooper
and Margaret Bamford

Blackwell Science Ltd
Editorial Offices:
Osney Mead, Oxford OX2 0EL
25 John Street, London WC1N 2BL
23 Ainslie Place, Edinburgh EH3 6AJ
238 Main Street, Cambridge,
    Massachusetts 02142, USA
54 University Street, Carlton,
    Victoria 3053, Australia

Other Editorial Offices:
Arnette Blackwell SA
224, Boulevard Saint Germain
75007 Paris, France

Blackwell Wissenschafts-Verlag GmbH
Kurfürstendamm 57
10707 Berlin, Germany

Zehetnergasse 6
A-1140 Wien
Austria

First published 1997

Set in 10 pt Century Book
by DP Photosetting, Aylesbury, Bucks
Printed and bound in Great Britain
by Hartnolls Ltd, Bodmin, Cornwall

The Blackwell Science logo is a trade mark
of Blackwell Science Ltd, registered at the
United Kingdom Trade Marks Registry.

DISTRIBUTORS

Marston Book Services Ltd
PO Box 269
Abingdon
Oxon OX14 4YN
(*Orders:* Tel: 01235 465500
        Fax: 01235 465555)

USA
Blackwell Science, Inc.
238 Main Street
Cambridge, MA 02142
(*Orders:* Tel: 800 215-1000
        617 876-7000
        Fax: 617 492-5263)

Canada
Copp Clark Professional
200 Adelaide Street, West, 3rd Floor
Toronto, Ontario M5H 1W7
(*Orders:* Tel: 416 597-1616
        800 815-9417
        Fax: 416 597-1617)

Australia
Blackwell Science Pty Ltd
54 University Street
Carlton, Victoria 3053
(*Orders:* Tel: 03 9347-0300
        Fax: 03 9347-5001)

A catalogue record for this title
is available from the British Library

ISBN 0-632-04032-7

Library of Congress
Cataloging-in-Publication Data

Excellence in health care management/
    edited by Alison Morton-Cooper and
    Margaret Bamford
        p. cm.
    Includes bibliographical references
    and index.
    ISBN 0-632-04032-7
    1. Health services administration.
    I. Morton-Cooper, Alison. II. Bamford,
    Margaret
    RA971.E986 1997
    362.1'068–dc20   96-21528
                                       CIP

Contents

List of Contributors

Margaret Bamford *PhD, MSc, RGN, DASTE, OHNC, DN Cert, Teaching Cert*
Consultant and Senior Research Fellow, University of Keele

Ann Close *MEd, BEd (Hons), RGN, RNT, DipN*
Nursing Director, Dudley Group of Hospitals NHS Trust

Christina Hughes *BA (Hons), PhD*
Lecturer, Department of Continuing Education, University of Warwick

Terry Hyland *PhD, MA, BEd, Cert Ed*
Lecturer in Continuing Education, University of Warwick

Sue Lillyman *MA, BSc, RGN, RM, DPSN, PGCE (FAHE)*
Nurse Lecturer, Personal Development Centre, Faculty of Health and Social Sciences, University of Central England, Birmingham

Alison Morton-Cooper *MEd, RGN*
Research Fellow, Centre for Continuing Education, University of Edinburgh

Carol Ward *RGN, DipN, DMS*
Management Consultant, Ward-Whitfield Associates, Stourbridge, West Midlands

Foreword

Excellence in Health Care Management fills a void in the literature for a text that addresses the more strategic, conceptual and thought-provoking issues of key health care debates, and helps students of management and information management, no matter what profession, to get to grips with these issues.

Nursing and the nursing service can no longer be seen in splendid isolation; the knowledgeable practitioner needs to explore issues that impact on the direct delivery of health care as we know it today and ask the question 'What do we want nursing to be in the future?' This has been the subject of discussions, conferences, seminars and published papers, with much rhetoric reflecting the idealised professional standards as the solution. Such answers, by dismissing any sense of realism, do little to enhance the status of nursing and merely deflect one from coping with the reality of resource limitations.

Nurses also have to explore where they, as professionals, fit into the scheme of things and re-examine their role in this changing world. The nursing process is slowly giving way to the patient process as healthcare professionals realise that individualised care has to be shared, not only between the professions, but more importantly with the individual for whom the service is intended.

How then are we to ensure that nurses are fully involved in developing the profession in a way that embraces these notions? The profession has to be in control of its own destiny, not only by being part of continuing professional development, but by ensuring that it is fully conversant with the possible future directions of training and the ways these may be funded.

There are literally thousands of management texts and the popular journals carry articles each week on health care management. Publishing collections of papers by different authors has become an increasingly popular method of attempting to pull together ideas of a similar nature in the same textbook and has at times resulted in boring and fragmented reading. I am grateful to the editors of this text who have had the wisdom to leave the authors to write in their own style, thus reflecting the authors' expertise and enthusiasm for the subject. *Excellence in Health Care Management* is an eminently readable text, which for the first time places a good collection of representative arguments in one place.

Graham Wright

Preface

This book is the conception of a group of people who wanted to fill the gap for an accessible introduction to the key issues and dilemmas facing health care managers today. The proliferation of management courses in health care is a necessary response to the need for managers at all levels to establish a legitimate place for themselves within the traditionally professionally-dominated context of health care. Here in the United Kingdom, a welfare state which was originally charged with eradicating the 'five giant evils' of Want, Ignorance, Squalor, Disease and Idleness has grown into a professionalised bureaucracy responsible for determining and meeting the needs of many with limited financial resources, and as such it has engendered a great deal of argument as to its legitimate uses and viability as a form of social organisation.

The so-called rise of managerialism as a counter-measure to the prevailing power of health professionals has led to many changes in practice and philosophy which we feel deserve closer and considered examination, rather than continuing disparagement and cries of despair. In the editors' view, the ciriticism currently levelled at managers may be a symptom of the more general malaise affecting staff attempting to provide a comprehensive and sensitive health care service within an (all too often) culture of negativism, and at times, despondency. In reality, the apparent intellectual crisis in health care provision probably cuts much deeper than the internecine warfare that has come to characterise relationships between health professionals and some of their manager colleagues. In the search for pragmatic solutions to our collective problems, we hope that the contributions included in this text will provide some useful background and contextual information which may then be used collaboratively to inform management practice. Given the burning need to develop theory *with* practice (and vice versa) contributors include practising managers, academics and educationalists in equal measure.

Each of the contributions was commissioned because of the apparent dearth of information on that subject experienced by our own students and colleagues. Arbitrary choices of academic levels do not inform the chapters, as we felt this would be too prescriptive. Rather, we hope that readers will be able to access the material at the level of their particular interest; as managers, students of health care and social policy, clinicians, educators, social or management theorists, human resource specialists, policy developers and planners. We have made no attempt at homogeneity either in writing style or philosophy of approach, but instead we hope to reflect the diverse nature of current opinion in meeting present day challenges and aspirations to excellence in care provision. Our intention is to focus and stimulate debate and contention regarding the various issues, and to signpost the beginner as well as the advanced student of health care management and policy to supporting sources of literature.

On behalf of the contributors we hope that at the very least some debate will continue as a consequence of dipping into and reading the various contributions. As the late Anthony Burgess' notable translation of Rostand's *Cyrano de Bergerac* courageously claimed, we hope to be 'the diamond in the ash of the ultimate combustion' that represents best practice in health care management. Whether we will succeed in developing health care management as a formally recognised discipline in its own right here in the UK (or whether we will simply spontaneously combust in the attempt!) is probably a matter for others' conjecture.

Alison Morton-Cooper and Margaret Bamford

Part I
EXCELLENCE IN HUMAN RESOURCE MANAGEMENT

1
Organisational Change: Implications for Human Resource Management

Christina Hughes

Introduction

Have a nice day!

The machine on the wall hands out numbered tickets to customers to mark their places in the queue. The reception staff are dressed in a uniform of blue striped shirts and plain blue skirts. As they find each customer's file and direct them to the waiting area they say that the waiting time should be no more than ten minutes. In the waiting area the plants and cushioned seats give an air of tranquil gentility. Whilst waiting, customers are frequently visited by staff to be informed of the progress of their visit. The level of service and courtesy would rival any top hotel.

As an National Health Service (NHS) customer I was impressed by the 'service' that I received when I recently took my daughter to the local NHS dental hospital. As a sociologist I was intrigued at the parallels evident in receiving dental care and purchasing consumer goods. The ticket machine was the same as that used at the deli in the local supermarket. The uniforms were reminiscent of those worn by hotel receptionists. The atmosphere was relaxed yet informative. It was clear to me that changes, witnessed albeit at this relatively superficial level, had happened in this dental hospital since my last visit some 20 years ago.

Those who work for the NHS do not need me to say that such changes go beyond the cosmetic. The NHS and Community Care Act of 1990, underwritten by New Right philosophy, has introduced major quasi-market developments (Glennerster & Le Grand 1995; Le Grand & Bartlett 1993). Indeed, the list of changes is seemingly endless. Purchaser/provider relationships, compulsory competitive tendering, performance appraisal, league tables, the growth of managerialism, customer orientation, quality assurance systems, installation of comprehensive resource management systems, the creation of Trusts and GP fund-holding, mergers and acquisitions. It is perhaps banal to say that turbulence is a way of life for those working in the NHS as in the public sector more generally (Painter 1991). Yet whilst change may be all around us, how might we make some sense of it?

In their analysis of such changes, Stewart and Walsh comment that they 'can be seen as attempts to change the cultures of the public services, dominated as they have been by the traditions of administration, hierarchy and professionalism' (Stewart & Walsh 1992, p. 508). This changing culture is, as Taylor-Gooby (1996) reminds us, set against the highly politicised nature of the 1990s reforms. Human resource professionals in the health sector not only have to be wary of importing oversimplified models from the private sector but also have to recognise the value base of the public domain (Stewart & Walsh 1992).

Discussions of culture and culture change are manifest in the literature on management theory and practice. Connections were made in the early 1980s by management gurus such as Peters and Waterman (1982) between creating the 'right' culture and organisational excellence. This has, however, usually been portrayed in a simplistic fashion (Wilson 1992). This chapter will attempt to avoid prescription and recipes. Rather, the position taken is that what is important is understanding and reflection on the various ways of seeing and knowing what the literature, and experience, has to offer.

Accordingly, the chapter will begin with a discussion of the ways in which the role of the human resource professional has shifted to an emphasis on being both a strategist and a manager of chaos. Here, the advent of post-modern theories of fragmentation vies with the universalism of institutional authority. The second section focuses on organisational culture, and considers whether culture can be defined at all. Associated change models form the basis of discussion in the third section. The message here has to do with the significance of recognising the association between one's operational understanding of culture and the mechanisms for change which are commonly instituted. The fourth section discusses the implications of change for individuals. It is perhaps within such a focus that the issue of values and ethics is most clear. The concluding section recalls aspects of professionality as key approaches for those who wish to cope, survive and perhaps develop within changing environments.

Changing terminologies, changing theories

Human resource management (HRM) is a relatively new concept to organisational theory. Introduced in the 1980s, along with its companion human resource development (HRD), it has, in many instances, displaced the terms personnel and training. The significance of this changing terminology lies in the ways in which conceptions of the role of those concerned with the administration of employment law, welfare, training and employee relations have shifted to a much greater focus on the strategic importance of HRM practices and policies as central to organisational survival and success.

This reorientation, from the micro issues of worker performance to the more macro concerns of organisational policy and direction, has led to a redefining of role and function for the human resource manager. Strategic human resource management (SHRM) is not confined to the preserves of a separate department dealing with day-to-day issues. As Martell and Carroll (1995) indicate, SHRM can be characterised as having a longer term focus. It is linked to organisational strategic planning, often at board or chief executive level, with a greater accountability for proving its contribution to economic performance.

This discovery of the importance of HRM/SHRM (and their associated term HRD) to organisational success takes as its unquestionable focus the development of the human capital potentiality of employees. Storey's (1995) definition makes the connections between strategy and people clear:

'Human resource management is a distinctive approach to employment management which seeks to achieve competitive advantage through the strategic deployment of a highly committed and capable workforce, using an integrated array of cultural, structural and personnel techniques.'

(Storey 1995, p. 5)

Integral to this position is the view that an organisation's only significant competitive advantage lies in its employees. People are not replicable in the ways that other resources, such as technology, materials or plant, are. Any competitor organisation can acquire such hardware. How they work it, however, depends on their employees. Accordingly, investment in the human resource is seen to be repayable in balance sheet terms and people are, within this perspective, a prized possession. They can provide the creative energy required to enhance productivity, find new markets, problem solve and enhance organisational capability.

Much work related to harnessing the creative capacity of the individual tends, however, to neglect the power dimensions inherent in the employment relationship. Writing in the field of the learning organisation provides classic examples where the positive connotations associated with the term suggest an unexamined 'win-win' for employer and employee, manager and managed (Hughes & Tight 1995; Tight 1996). Nevertheless, Townley's (1994) acknowledgement of the relationship between HRM and power and knowledge addressed in a Foucauldian analysis reasserts the importance of recognising the politics and ethics of work. Rather than an apolitical arbiter of policy, attention is drawn to the way in which HRM practices 'create order and knowledge, and through this produce a technology of power' (Townley 1994, p. 20).

The changing conceptions of employee management encompassed within the terms HRM/SHRM represent one strand in restating the role of the human resource professional. An associated strand is the development of theories of organisational life which reject the techno-rational orientations found within Tayloristic and Fordist views where tasks are broken into components for managing the production process. Organisation theory now places considerable emphasis on understanding organisations as ambiguous, multi-reality sites where, paradoxically, control is exercised through the acceptance of the uncontrollable nature of many facets of organisational life.

The changing orientation of organisational theory can be summarised in relatively simple comparative statements as Lannon (1996) indicates. For example, within post-modernist understandings there is a questioning of institutional authority and an emphasis on egalitarianism and individualism. This can be compared with the suggestions of stability, hierarchy and inherited values to be found in the early industrial era.

Alternatively, the use of metaphor for indicating the multiple ways in which organisations can be analysed and understood inevitably questions those who promulgate universal conceptions. Morgan (1986) provides perhaps the classic statement of the metaphorical position where among the eight metaphors for understanding organisational life listed are organisations as instruments of domination, as psychic prisons, as brains *and* as cultures.

The equivocal, even cryptic, nature of how we might understand what an organisation is, encompassed within Morgan's metaphors, conveys a central element of current theory. Such ambiguity is the concept which summarises understandings of organisational life. Tsoukas (1994) identifies four sources of ambiguity which belie any concept of rational ordered organisation. These are that:

'organisations are often unclear what their intentions are; they do not know unequivocally what is appropriate for them to do; they are usually unable to identify exactly what they did in the past and why; and it is not always clear who in the organisation is responsible for what.'

(Tsoukas 1994, p. 11).

Yet, if organisations are marked by ambiguity, defining culture carries the same difficulties.

Developing cultural analysis

The ephemeral nature of conceptualising, let alone concretising, the notion of culture is evident in any review of the organisational literature. Wright's statement that 'Culture has acquired multifarious meanings in the literature on organisations' (Wright 1994, p. 17) is indeed succinct. Wilson (1992) avoids defining culture precisely because there are so many definitions in the literature and because it is used in such an all-encompassing way. Culture is a slippery word and this is where its influence lies. Its varied definitional status lends itself to usage by diverse interest groups and distinct political and philosophical perspectives.

It is important to recognise that these different ways of seeing and understanding what culture is will inform the frameworks and recommendations embedded in change programmes. In a review of the literature on culture and cultural change Meyerson and Martin (1994) identify three paradigmatic approaches: integration, differentiation and ambiguity. Caution should be exercised, however, in viewing these positions as mutually exclusive and static as there are areas of overlap or transfer of ideas.

Newman indicates that 'organisational culture' is usually defined in terms of shared symbols, language, practices ('how we do things around here'), and 'deeply embedded beliefs and values' (Newman, 1995, p. 11). The first, and indeed the most common, paradigm identified by Meyerson and Martin (1994) is that of 'integration'. This emphasis on consensus and shared beliefs has a tendency to consider culture as monolithic and consensual. It is encompassed within terms such as 'the company culture'. The creators of culture, within this perspective, are company leaders and in any analysis of organisational culture the statements of senior management and their translation would be significant.

The integrationist perspective is useful in its recognition of the power and influence of those at the top as architects of working environments. Many companies, including GKN, Cadbury Schweppes, Rowntree Mackintosh, British Steel and British Airways, have made explicit statements of their culture (Wilson & Rosenfeld 1990). However, the focus on unity and being 'as one' implicit in this position can neglect the diversity and combative nature of values and beliefs. It can also forget that organisations are as much political systems as cultural ones. As Morgan states, 'in organisations there are often many different and competing value systems that create a mosaic of organisational realities rather than a uniform corporate culture' (Morgan, 1986, p. 127). Thus Meyerson and Martin (1994) identify 'differentiation' as their second paradigm.

The spotlight within differentiation perspectives of culture is placed on sub-groups and sub-cultures. Sub-cultures may arise from different professional groupings, classes, genders, ethnicities and so forth. Key elements of this position are the emphasis given to the contradictions in values found in the workplace and the ways in which organisational practices are not necessarily the same as espoused values. Rather than consensus, as found in an integrationist view, this approach stresses the potentiality of disagreement between bounded groups. Accordingly, a top-down view from the perspective of senior executives would not be the sole investigative position of the cultural analyst but would form only part of the research framework. Rather the focus would be on identifying the range of sub-cultures within the organisation.

The strength of differentiation perspectives lies in the recognition of a plurality of cultures. Feminist work on the gendered nature of organisational environments provides examples of the use of this position (see for example Itzin & Newman 1995; Shaw & Perrons 1995; Tanton 1994). The association of management with masculine styles of behaviour (Limerick & Lingard 1995) and the analysis of barriers such as paper, rubber and glass ceilings (Stamp 1995) suggest the importance of sub-cultural dimensions.

Work in relation to national cultures can be seen as a further example of the sub-cultural position. In this instance, however, the organisation itself is viewed as the differentiated object. The findings of commentators such as Hofstede (1980, 1993, 1996) imply the significance for human resource professionals of understanding national cultures, particularly for the global firm. International understandings of the practices and meanings of management provide an illustration. In North America and the United Kingdom management is perceived both as a procedure and as a class of people. Managers act on behalf of owners, or the state, to motivate other employees to produce goods and services. A round-robin tour of the developed world might indicate alternative understandings of management. For example, in Germany the role of the meister as expert is to resolve technical problems and allocate tasks. In Japan, control is exerted by peer group rather than manager. In China, familial connections provide the bedrock of business with decision making in the hands of one dominant family member (Hofstede 1996).

From this viewpoint adapting to local cultural conditions is a prerequisite for success (Smith 1992). Attention to the significance of national culture also points out one of the problems of importing policies and practices from other countries. As those seeking to *Japanise* have found, not taking sufficient account of the cultural contexts in which such policies and practices were developed can lead to failure.

While integration and differentiation, as concepts, imply oppositional positions, they nevertheless share commonalities. Differentiation shares with integration an assumption of shared values whether this is at the level of sub-group, organisation or nation. Women, ethnic groups, professionals, classes, nations and so forth are assumed to be distinctive groupings. Part of their distinctiveness is an assumption that members of each group think, and behave, alike. This view clearly leads to the creation of stereotypes and the likelihood of understanding individual, organisation and nation as closed systems. Developments in understandings of the concept of difference and within post-modernist thinking indicate that such assumptions are problematic (Nicholson 1990).

As within organisation theory more generally, work in relation to organisational cultures is beginning to take account of post-modernist thought, in particular through the concept of ambiguity. This term in fact forms the third paradigmatic approach identified by Meyerson and Martin (1994). Whereas the descriptions of integration and differentiation suggest, either at the level of the organisation as a whole or through the existence of sub-groups, boundaries around groups according to their shared norms and values, ambiguity approaches the understanding of culture with a view which states that:

> 'individuals share some viewpoints, disagree about some, and are ignorant of or indifferent to others. Consensus, dissensus, and confusion coexist, making it difficult to draw cultural and subcultural boundaries.'
>
> (Meyerson & Martin 1994, pp. 122–3)

This approach to cultural analysis highlights fragmentation, fluidity and contradiction within individual value positions. It draws attention to the problems of placing boundaries around categories and leads to a focus on language and power, discourse and identity as essential to understanding organisations. Foucauldian analyses, for example, would reject ideas that personnel practices can only be effective when they are less subjective and more accurate (Townley 1994). Townley argues that:

> 'The individual is not a "given", essential identity but is actively produced. One mechanism for this is to construct the individual as an object of knowledge and power.'
>
> (Townley 1994, p. 83)

This individualistic position is, nevertheless, problematic as it attracts attention away from the structural. In addition, taken to its ultimate conclusion it negates the very concepts of culture and of organisation. As Olie (1995) indicates, a defining element of culture is that it is 'not a characteristic of individuals, but of a collection of individuals who share common values, beliefs, ideas' (Olie 1995, p. 127). For those concerned with organisational change, the degree of sharedness is clearly important.

McDonaldise or self-organise? Choices in organisational change strategies

In a study focused on responses to the development of the internal market in the NHS, Dent (1995) examined issues of managerial vs. professional autonomy and control. Working from the findings of Ritzer (1993) in the United States of America, Dent was interested in whether new forms of bureaucratic control would be put into effect which would 'McDonaldise' the Health Service. The emphasis within the McDonald-isation thesis is on standardisation and demarcated tasks, taking Taylorist and Fordist principles of work organisation into the post-modern era.

Dent's findings concur with those of Calnan and Williams (1995) in respect of the malleability of medical autonomy. Dent argued that what he found was not a process of McDonaldization but re-professionalisation. 'Doctors have suffered nothing worse than a comfortable incorporation with the new system as senior managers' (Dent 1995, p. 894). Dent places his analysis within a post-modern approach to organisational analysis. He argues that hospital management:

'were intent on adapting and developing their own autonomy and flexibility [in a culture which] was used politically to integrate ... complex and fragmentary relational forms.'

(Dent 1995, p. 895)

Dent's work is instructive as an example of the lenses by which we might understand change. McDonaldisation as a process suggests the imposition or creation of a strong company culture, the integrated voice of the organisation. Dent's findings suggest the existence of a culture of professional autonomy, the differentiated voice of a sub-group. Yet to survive, this sub-group has to be environmentally adaptive. It does so through negotiating the, often unarticulated, ambiguities of organisational life.

All of these positions imply their own approaches to how change might be enacted. Schein (1992) gives us the clearest statement that those who can effect cultural change are those who occupy the senior positions in organisations. 'Leaders ... create and modify cultures. Culture creation, culture evolution, and culture management are what ultimately define leadership' (Schein 1992, p. xv). Change therefore can be enacted through new mission or vision statements or the espousal of new values by top management. The concomitant process is described in three stages (Schein 1992, pp. 298 ff). To create the motivation to change, the first stage requires the 'unfreezing' of old attitudes and behaviours. Stage two requires that new behaviours, values and meanings are learned through a process of 'cognitive restructuring'. As the name indicates, 'refreezing' at stage three suggests that once in place the new world-view remains safe and unquestioned. Until, of course, further change is required.

For Meyerson and Martin (1994) Schein's work is the classic statement of those who occupy the integrationist paradigm. It assumes the collapse of one total company view to be replaced, through manipulation, by another. This perspective within the cultural change literature is the most common and fits within assumptions that culture is a 'lever' which can be mechanistically pulled (Morgan 1986; Newman 1995). Its attraction is the promise of a quick-fix through the control that can seemingly be exercised by those at the top of organisations.

Whilst discord needs to be eliminated for those who present a one-world view of culture, for others it can represent an important ally. As Pemberton indicates 'For those working in equalities departments the creation of a subculture may be absolutely necessary to sustain motivation, self-confidence, and group identity' (Pemberton 1995, p. 116). Yet whilst sub-groups can form support networks and cohesion, the politics of, and resistance to, change is more manifest for those who are interested in challenging dominant views.

> 'Difference(s) from others are frequently about forming and maintaining group boundaries. The brutal and bloody nature of this maintenance work is everywhere in evidence.'
>
> (Moore 1994, p. 1)

The acknowledgement of sub-cultures and their role in the change process represents a less optimistic view of change strategies. One might say a less utopian view. The locus of control is not so easy to identify and, rather than offering the potential of a total remodelling, change is likely to be incremental and diffuse giving rise to intended and unintended consequences. As Guest *et al.* (1993) indicate in a study of employee involvement in part of British Rail, training designed to change 'Them' and 'Us' attitudes did not result in any wholesale reidentification with management views. However, there was evidence of some shift towards a more local pattern of identity which excluded union representatives from the 'Us'.

Whilst sub-cultural understandings of change signify diversity and a lowering of control by those who perceive themselves as change agents, within post-modernist theory the potential for control is reduced still further. Indeed, within frames of reference which stress:

'a recovery of the notions of *chaos* [emphasis in text], chance, luck and the indeterminable as an integral part of organisational behaviour and the societies in which we live'

(Cummings 1996, p. 261)

the exercise of control becomes impossible. Change is continual, acting upon and being enacted by organisational members to the extent that if a locus of control exists it lies within the individual (Meyerson & Martin 1994).

Underlying this view is the idea that organisations cannot be understood in terms of fixed, objective realities. Rather organisations are viewed as collections of individuals who, through a process of reflection, are engaged in making constant interpretations of their social reality. Accordingly, the process of 'organising' becomes the principle through which organisation is understood. Viewing organisation in these terms implicitly holds, as the only certainty, the existence of flux and flow. Prediction becomes more difficult as one cannot know with any assurance how individuals might interpret the changes around them.

This is clearly not a perspective for those who prefer ordered conceptions of social reality or who feel safer with high levels of predictability. Nevertheless, given that levels of ambiguity are highest in organisations whose concerns are people-centred, such as health, welfare and educational services (Meyerson & Martin 1994; Tsoukas 1994), and where many staff are professionalised, there is a case here for those who seek a 'best fit' approach between type of organisation and change strategy. Recognising the potential value of this process leads to a pattern of organisation which is itself constantly changing. The rationale underlying organisation, for example, would be issue-based with individuals working together, reforming or reordering as appropriate. To facilitate this process clearly considerable individual autonomy is required.

This focus on the individual leads us into extending our organisational perspectives into a more intrepretivist view. As Wilson notes, the interpretive approach asks the personal question 'What will the changes mean for me?' (Wilson 1992, p. 82).

Confronting apprehension? Organisational change for individuals

It is open to debate whether the level or extent of changes being experienced in all areas of public service are unprecedented (Tight 1995). For example, Imershein and Estes' (1996) work in respect of health reforms in the United States of America views current reforms as a second stage in the development of non-profit organisations within capitalist economies. In respect of the British Health Service, reminders of the development of health services at the turn of the century, and perhaps more particularly of the changes associated with the Beveridge reforms of 1948, reawaken an important sense of historical perspective. Nevertheless, for the individual encountering or being subjected to change, the experience may be new, unexpected, unwanted and filled with anxiety.

The effect of increasing work loads and insecurity, inherent within cultures focused on efficiency gains, can give rise to higher levels of stress and harassment at work (Incomes Data Services 1996). Indeed, the associations between working conditions and mental health are beginning to be recognised in case law. In 1995, *Walker* v *Northumberland County Council* was the first case where an employee succeeded in establishing such connections. The implications for human resource professionals are manifest. From the human resource perspective, as Iverson notes, whilst change is everywhere 'the one thing that has remained the same is the requirement of employees to adapt to organisational change' (Iverson 1996, p. 122).

Iverson's research focused on the introduction of market forces in a public hospital in Australia. His purpose was to develop a causal model which would enable organisations to predict the level of employee acceptance to change. Using a survey approach, Iverson asked a range of questions across three main variables. These were: personal, including union membership, age, education, sex, tenure, occupation; job-related, including autonomy, job security, promotional opportunity, job ambiguity and role conflict; and environmental, including industrial relations climate and kinship responsibility.

Whilst Iverson argued for a multi-faceted approach to change, overall his findings concur with those of Guest (1995) and suggest that 'organisational commitment should be considered as a determinant, as well as a mediator of factors in the change process' (Iverson 1996, p. 143). Iverson urges human resource policies to be focused on encouraging organisational commitment and loyalty. In an era which heralds the flexible workforce as the centre-piece of human resource planning, fostering allegiance can become an act of creativity in itself.

Kanter (1989, 1996) draws our attention to the inherent tensions between corporate flexibility and individual security. As she states:

'Businesses want and need the flexibility to restructure, to change shape, and to pursue new streams, while employees want the security of knowing there is a place for them.'

(Kanter 1996, p. 52)

To achieve this conjuring trick, Kanter emphasises the importance of finding individual security through employability.

Individuals, Kanter argues, need to develop four related skills if they are to enhance their employability. These relate to a belief in self rather than the power of one's position; the ability to collaborate and work with teams; a commitment to the intrinsic excitement of achievement in a particular project; and a willingness to keep learning (Kanter 1989, pp. 364–5). Accordingly, individuals build their career through an investment in their own personal capital rather than through accumulating organisational capital by mechanisms such as length of service.

The model outlined by Kanter stresses the individualist position. It is matched by an equally strong emphasis in current writing on organisational competitiveness which encourages flexible employment strategies. Yet, there is 'much more stable employment around than the pundits would have us believe' (Incomes Data Services 1995, p. 5). Whilst flexibility has advantages 'it is hard to avoid the impression that this is often a modern disguise for some very old-fashioned types of employment' (Incomes Data Services 1995, p. 15). Indeed, whilst flexibility may be 'new wine in old bottles' (Pollert, 1991), there is no doubt that companies are rediscovering the value of stable, permanent employment in terms of its contribution to organisational effectiveness.

From the viewpoint of human resource strategy one of the problems with employing 'flexible' workers relates not only to the need for organisational commitment but also to ensuring that workers have relevant, and up-to-date, skills and knowledge. Mandatory requirements for the continuing professional development of nursing staff provide one area where the tensions around 'who pays' when staff are casualised become evident. In many sectors of employment, the inherent costs of training, and consequently maintaining employability when in 'flexible' employment, are being passed on to individuals (Department of Employment 1995). Recognising the mutuality embedded in the values of loyalty and commitment appears to be a key human resource skill which is currently absent in far too many workplaces.

The work of Iverson and Kanter is written from a more sociological perspective than psychological. Their work emphasises the structural rather than the emotional. Yet a listing of the defence mechanisms which individuals commonly exhibit when they face change draws attention to the importance of the psychological. Repression, regression, projection, reaction formation and denial have all been found as responses to change (Vince & Broussine 1996).

As everyday reactions, Vince and Broussine (1996) argue that these defence processes should be acknowledged rather than ignored in the change process. By focusing on role boundaries and managers' implicit understandings of boundaries between groups in the workplace, Vince and Broussine's research encouraged managers in six public service organisations to understand the relational and emotional contexts in which organisational change operates. They suggest that there are four stages to encouraging an enhanced attention to the emotional.

First, managers need to stay with uncertainty long enough not to automatically deny or avoid the feelings associated with it. Second, rather than seeing the boundaries between groups as clearer than they actually are, managers need to reflect on their assumptions about group identities and attachments. Third, managers need to develop a sense of the relatedness between emotionality and change in order that recognition of one's own emotions associated with change can promote tolerance. Finally, stage four requires mechanisms for working together to be found so that the changes can be worked through.

It is interesting that Vince and Broussine, like Schein, suggest a linear, staged process to deal with, as they acknowledge, the complex and ambiguous aspects of organisation. Nevertheless, just as managing creativity requires attention to some down-to-earth issues such as pay and opportunities for professional recognition (Incomes Data Services 1994), psychological safety in periods of change may similarly be enhanced through an understanding of the frameworks of change themselves. To return to Meyerson and Martin's paradigms outlined earlier, as markers of how things are changing, new mission statements can provide an important element of clarity. Or sub-groups may provide protective dens by mediating the impact of wider organisational change. When change is ever present, the encouragement of autonomy can bring its own sense of safety (Meyerson & Martin 1994). For the human resource professional, the development of one's personal sense of autonomy is implicit in the growth of their professionality.

Professionality: Concluding reflections on change

This chapter has presented a variety of approaches to the question of managing change. These include viewing organisations as single entities, as a mix of competing sub-groups and as comprised of the subjectivity of individuals. The perspectives brought to understanding what an organisation is, or indeed how it should be, can be associated with different change strategies or models. Top down, bottom up, empowerment and autonomy are common examples. The individual view reasserts a focus on the connections between the changing structures of employment and employment practices and their potential effects for personal well-being. But a final important question remains. What can the human resource professional, living with constant change, do to contribute to their own empowerment?

One thing is clear. The organisation is contestable space, from theoretical, practice and values viewpoints. For organisational changers, becoming adept at multiple 'readings' of organisational life is requisite. Reflective practice, well known in the literature related to the ways in which professionality can be developed, would appear an obvious route to such adeptness (Argyris & Schön, 1976; Schön, 1983, 1988). In essence, and with the aim of improvement in mind, such reflection requires the professional to critically reflect and to evaluate their performance.

The attractiveness of the concept of the reflective practitioner, however, lies not only in the potential for enhanced performance but also in the emphasis given to the skills of critical reflection. Here, a range of conceptual and theoretical frameworks, importantly including an understanding of one's own, are brought to the processes of explanation and understanding. It is not surprising that a similar emphasis on multiple explanation, and the associated range of potential solutions, is also associated with the development of expertise (Benner 1984; Chi *et al.* 1988). Indeed, we might conclude by suggesting that becoming an expert at both personal and organisational change is an important trait for human resource professionals. In essence, finding creative routes to such expertise is what change should be about.

References

Argyris, C. & Schon, D. (1976) *Theory in Practice: Increasing Professional Effectiveness.* Jossey Bass, San Francisco.
Benner, P. (1984) *From Novice to Expert: Excellence and Power in Clinical Nursing.* Addison-Wesley, Menlo Park, CA.
Calnan, M. & Williams, S. (1995) Challenges to professional autonomy in the United Kingdom? The perceptions of General Practitioners, *International Journal of Health Services,* **25**(2), 219–41.
Chi, M., Glaser, R. & Farr, M. (eds) (1988) *The Nature of Expertise.* Laurence Erlbaum Associates, Hillsdale, NJ.
Cummings, S. (1996) Back to the oracle: post-modern organization theory as resurfacing of pre-modern wisdom. *Organization,* **3**(2), 249–66.

Dent, M. (1995) The new National Health Service: a case of postmodernism?. *Organization Studies*, **16**(5), 875–99.

Department of Employment (1995) *Labour Market and Skills Trends 1994–95*. Skills and Enterprise Network, Nottingham.

Guest, D., Peccei, R. & Thomas, A. (1993) The impact of employee involvement on organisational commitment and 'them and us' attitudes. *Industrial Relations*, **31**(2), 191–200.

Guest, D.E. (1995) Human Resource Management, Trade Unions and Industrial Relations. In: *Human Resource Management: A Critical Text* (ed. J. Storey), pp. 110–41. Routledge, London.

Glennerster, H. & Le Grand, J. (1995) The development of quasi-markets in welfare provision in the United Kingdom. *International Journal of Health Services*, **25**(2), 203–18.

Hofstede, G. (1980) *Culture's Consequences: International Differences in Work-related Values*. Sage, London.

Hofstede, G. (1993) Cultural constraints in management theories. *Academy of Management Executive*, **7**(1), 81–93.

Hofstede, G. (1996) A shrinking world: cultural constraints in management theories. In: *The New Management Reader* (eds R. Paton, G. Clark, G. Jones, J. Lewis & P. Quintas), pp. 77–90. Routledge/Open University, London.

Hughes, C. & Tight, M. (1995) The myth of the learning society. *British Journal of Educational Studies*, **43**(3), 290–304.

Imershein, A.W. & Estes, C.L. (1996) From health services to medical markets: the commodity transformation of medical production and the nonprofit sector. *International Journal of Health Services*, **26**(2), 221–38.

Incomes Data Services (1994) Managing creativity. *IDS Focus 73*, Incomes Data Services Limited, London.

Incomes Data Services (1995) The jobs mythology. *IDS Focus 74*, Incomes Data Services Limited, London.

Incomes Data Services (1996) Bullying and harassment at work. *IDS Employment Law Supplement 76*, Incomes Data Services Limited, London.

Itzin, C. & Newman, J. (1995) *Gender, Culture and Organizational Change: Putting Theory into Practice*. Routledge, London.

Iverson, R.D. (1996) Employee acceptance of organizational change: the role of organizational commitment. *International Journal of Human Resource Management*, **7**(1), 122–49.

Kanter, R.M. (1989) *When Giants Learn to Dance*. Routledge, London.

Kanter, R.M. (1996) Beyond the cowboy and the corpocrat. In: *How Organizations Learn* (ed. K. Starkey), pp. 43–59. International Thomson Business Press, London.

Lannon, J. (1996) Mosaics of meaning: anthropology and marketing. In: *The New Management Reader* (eds R. Paton, G. Clark, G. Jones, J. Lewis & P. Quintas), pp. 23–40. Routledge/Open University, London.

Le Grand, J. & Bartlett, W. (eds) (1993) *Quasi-Markets and Social Policy*. MacMillan, London.

Limerick, B. & Lingard, B. (eds) (1995) *Gender and Changing Educational Management*. Hodder Education, Rydalmere (NSW).

Martell, K. & Carroll, S.J. (1995) How strategic is HRM? *Human Resource Management*, **34**(2), 253–67.

Meyerson, D. & Martin, J. (1994) Cultural change: an integration of three different views. In: *New Thinking in Organizational Behaviour* (ed. H. Tsoukas), pp. 108–32. Butterworth-Heinemann, Oxford.

Moore, H. (1994) *A Passion for Difference*. Polity, Cambridge.

Morgan, G. (1986) *Images of Organization*. Sage, Newbury Park, CA.

Newman, J. (1995) Gender and cultural change. In: *Gender, Culture and Organizational Change: Putting Theory into Practice* (eds C. Itzin & J. Newman), pp. 11–29. Routledge, London.

Nicholson, L.J. (1990) *Feminism/Postmodernism*. Routledge, London.

Olie, R. (1995) The 'culture' factor in personnel and organization policies. In: *International Human Resource Management* (eds A. Wil Harzing & J.V. Ruysseveldt), pp. 124–43. Sage, London.

Painter, C. (1991) The public sector and current orthodoxies: revitalisation or decay? *Political Quarterly*, **62**(1), 79–89.

Pemberton, C. (1995) Organizational culture and equalities work. In: *Making Gender Work: Managing Equal Opportunities* (eds J. Shaw & D. Perrons), pp. 108–24. Open University Press, Buckingham.

Peters, T. & Waterman, R. (1982) *In Search of Excellence: Lessons from America's Best-run Companies*. Harper and Row, New York.

Pollert, A. (ed.) (1991) *Farewell to Flexibility?* Blackwell Publishers, Oxford.

Ritzer, G. (1993) *The McDonaldization of Society*. Pine Forge, Thousand Oaks, CA.

Schein, E.H. (1992) *Organizational Culture and Leadership*, 2nd edn. Jossey-Bass, San Francisco, CA.

Schön, D. (1983) *The Reflective Practitioner: How Professionals Think in Action*. Temple Smith, London.

Schön, D. (1988) *Educating the Reflective Practitioner*. Jossey-Bass, San Francisco, CA.

Shaw, J. & Perrons, D. (1995) *Making Gender Work: Managing Equal Opportunities*. Open University Press, Buckingham.

Smith, P.B. (1992) Organizational behaviour and national cultures. *British Journal of Management*, **3**, 39–51.

Stamp, G. (1995) The appeal and the claims of non-dominant groups. In: *Making Gender Work: Managing Equal Opportunities* (eds J. Shaw & D. Perrons), pp. 193–213. Open University Press, Buckingham.

Stewart, J. & Walsh, K. (1992) Change in the management of public services. *Public Administration*, **70**(3), 499–518.

Storey, J. (ed.) (1995) *Human Resource Management: A Critical Text*. Routledge, London.

Tanton, M. (ed.) (1994) *Women in Management: A Developing Presence*. Routledge, London.

Taylor-Gooby, P.I. (1996) The future of health care in six European countries: the views of policy elites. *International Journal of Health Services*, **26**(2), 203–19.

Tight, M. (1995) Crisis, what crisis? Rhetoric and reality in higher education. *British Journal of Educational Studies*, **42**(4), 363–74.

Tight, M. (1996) *Key Concepts in Adult Education and Training.* Routledge, London.

Townley, B. (1994) *Reframing Human Resource Management: Power, Ethics and the Subject at Work.* Sage, London.

Tsoukas, H. (ed.) (1994) *New Thinking in Organizational Behaviour.* Butterworth-Heinemann, Oxford.

Vince, R. & Broussine, M. (1996) Paradox, defence and attachment: accessing and working with emotions and relations underlying organisational change. *Organization Studies,* **17**(1), 1–22.

Wilson, D.C. (1992) *A Strategy of Change: Concepts and Controversies in the Management of Change.* Routledge, London.

Wilson, D. & Rosenfeld, R. (eds) (1990) *Managing Organisations.* McGraw Hill, London.

Wright, S. (1994) 'Culture' in anthropology and organization studies. In: *Anthropology of Organizations* (ed. S. Wright), pp. 1–31. Routledge, London.

2

Health Careers in the
Twenty-first Century

Margaret Bamford

What will constitute a health career in the twenty-first century? This chapter explains the issues surrounding criss-crossing role boundaries in health care. Dr Bamford analyses the nature of the contemporary workforce, its context and the underlying socio-political factors affecting human resource management policy in the health care sectors, but with a particular emphasis (given the author's experience and professional background) on the contribution to be made by nursing, midwifery and health visiting staff. As sociologist Anne Witz has observed:

'... in view of trends towards the decentralisation of health service finance and organisation, any global or collective vision of a nursing of the future is likely to be rapidly displaced by local variations in the health division of labour, within which the role of nurses will take shape, most probably in a largely pragmatic and ad hoc manner. It is increasingly likely, then, that the localised power of doctors and the new general managers will become more critical than in the past in shaping the possibility and direction of change in nursing, as well as the nature of work and power relations between doctors and nurses.'

(Witz 1994, p. 42)

The strategic importance of this issue ethically, logistically and economically is therefore one of central concern to health care managers involved in the distribution, rationing and logistical support of vital human resources. Dr Bamford places the priorities for service planning within a broader framework, drawing on recent developments in organisations as learning environments and in the restructuring of the workforce to meet perceived client needs.

Introduction

Nursing, midwifery and health visiting in the twenty-first century is an issue which has been exercising the minds of many people recently.

What will constitute a health career in the twenty-first century? There is concern that nursing as we know it will never be the same again (DoH 1993; RCN 1994). The concern is part of the general unease caused by the sweeping changes in the National Health Service (NHS) which seem to threaten the very foundation of nursing, midwifery and health visiting. This chapter will explore some of the issues surrounding the professional and managerial contribution of nursing, midwifery and health visiting, look at those issues against an organisational backdrop which is constantly changing and redefining its boundaries. There will increasingly be a blurring of these boundaries with multi-skilling, multi-faceted contributors to health care.

There is a strongly held view that nurses have not had a good level of morale since the mid-1980s (Robinson, J. 1992; Edwards 1993). The Griffiths NHS Management Inquiry Report (House of Commons (HoC) 1984) is often cited as the catalyst for nursing disenfranchisement from the NHS:

'Reports were emerging informally, and in the nursing press, of chief nursing officers at district and regional levels of the health service losing in some instances their jobs; in many cases their control over the nursing budget; and in others, their line management of nursing.'

(Robinson, J. 1992, p. 1)

The Griffiths Report, (HoC 1984) was an enquiry team established by the Secretary of State, and chaired by Mr Roy Griffiths, Managing Director of Sainsbury's. The team was to:

'give advice on the effective use and management of manpower and related resources in the NHS.'

(HoC 1984, p. vi)

It was proposed that the general management function should be met by a:

'type of chief executive who would be the ultimate decision taker, provide leadership, motivate staff, and ensure that the professional functions are effectively geared into the overall objectives and responsibilities of the general management function.'

(HoC 1984, p. xx)

General managers were to be placed at regional, district and unit level to move the NHS forward.

Edwards (1993) would argue that this was but one of a catalogue of incidents which saw the demise of nursing as we knew it. Factors contributing to this were: lack of professional identity; a traditional and authoritarian hierarchy, out of touch with modern women's views; inappropriate and diverse models to identify the nursing needs of dependent patients; emerging novel approaches to professional practice which were not supported wholeheartedly by the profession (the nursing process); new training approaches (Project 2000), and new and exciting roles for highly skilled practitioners. When set against the existing organisation turbulence it can be seen that a comfortable life was not on the agenda.

Robinson, J. (1992) describes a 'flash of insight' arrived at by herself and Phillip Strong in analysing their research findings. They felt that the Griffiths reforms were not about controlling nursing and implementing general management, but rather controlling medicine; and that nursing, which was 'invisible to virtually everyone except nurses' (p. 4), 'was merely caught in the crossfire' (p. 5). A very difficult position to be in!

Analysis of contemporary workforce

Celia Davies (1990) made public the concerns and anxieties felt by many people involved in nursing, midwifery and health visiting in her work for the English National Board (ENB). The earlier work by Charles Handy (1984; 1989) is the theoretical underpinning used by Davies. Handy (1984; 1989) argues that work as we knew it would change dramatically; full-time, life-long work would be a thing of the past. People would need to be not only more flexible in their approach to work, they would need to be more flexible in their thinking about work. This thinking might involve having one or two part-time jobs instead of one full-time job, perhaps working for more that one employer, or working from home. Davies (1990) felt that these changes occurring in society generally would also affect nursing. These changes are being reported in the press:

> 'There seem to be new reports of nurses facing redundancy almost weekly, newly qualified staff nurses looking at short and sometimes very short-term contracts, or the prospect of unemployment.'
>
> (Mangan 1994, p. 29)

In the 1980s it was anticipated that we were on the verge of a demographic time-bomb, that we would have insufficient new young workers entering the employment field to fill the vacancies left by the departing older workers (Mangan 1994). For a variety of reasons this did not happen at that time. During the late 1980s there were 'roughly half a million' nurses and midwives employed in the NHS in the UK (Robinson 1992). In the UK nearly half of the workforce is female, however, in nursing this rises to 90 per cent. A large proportion of these women work part time. Men in nursing held a disproportional number of higher grade posts in comparison to full-time female colleagues (Davies & Rosser 1986). So nursing, midwifery and health visiting are seen as feminine occupations with all the social and economic implications that this infers, such as low pay, low esteem, limited power (Salvage 1992).

Perhaps we need to take a hard look at how nurses have been used in the past. Many student nurses over the past 20 to 30 years were used primarily as an important part of the labour force, their contribution to delivering health care was considerable. In some instances education and training needs came secondary to service commitment. A cynical view would be that the unskilled level of contribution was what was needed, and that if there was a steady trickle of leavers during the three-year period, it could be met by increasing student numbers or the frequency of student intake. If newly qualified staff also sought other employment it would not be too big a problem.

Problems of staffing occurring at different levels, for example highly technical care areas, would however, elicit a different response. (Moccia 1990). The education and training lead-in time is much longer, and the investment much greater: what is to be done? Take experienced staff from another employer? This flow of staff is manageable in times of full employment, however, in a recession a different response is evoked. People are more anxious about moving job, particularly if their partner is unemployed, and then gaps in the system occur. These gaps have to be filled, service still has to be delivered.

Manpower planning in the NHS has never been an exact science, and this is not specific to the UK (Abdellah 1990; Moccia 1990). In the United States both these authors identify a constant and persistent shortage of nurses since the mid-1940s, and this is despite strong professional and governmental support, initiatives and developments. The recession in the UK has resulted in a smaller turnover of staff in recent years. In many families the women have been the main bread winners; the demise of masculine work, retrenchment of the industrial base, and removal of unskilled traditional male work have all worked toward this outcome. Women who work in the NHS have naturally been loathe to leave jobs with established contracts of employment. This has had a short-term effect of changing employment patterns, and encouraging planners and managers to feel confident about their manpower plans.

Project 2000 will address some of the education, training and employment issues facing students of nursing and midwifery. The demographic black hole predicted in the 1980s has probably not been so noticeable because of the rapid cut back in student numbers and the opening of access to training for non-traditional entrants. Conversion programmes for enrolled nurses will also have filled the gap to some extent. These changes bring with them a consideration of what the future of nursing is, and what will be attractive as a health career in the twenty-first century (Donovan 1990; Moccia 1990; van Maanen 1990).

Health careers in the twenty-first century

The issues need to be seen in context. Perhaps the question could be asked about whose context, but initially let us start with a fairly broad brush! In 1992, the Welsh Health Planning Forum (WHPF) sub-group produced a paper entitled *Health and Social Care 2010*, (WHPF 1992). Their intention was to produce a set of assumptions which could be piloted to produce a 'sensible health care delivery framework'. This work would then be moved on, through revision, to produce a strategic intent for Wales. This paper then went on to identify some benchmarks for the year 2002.

'The chosen assumptions are:
* by 2002, targets on smoking, physical exercise and weight are met
* for each local community there should be arrangements for pooling NHS and local authority funds to provide local access to
  ○ minor surgery
  ○ a minor accident service
  ○ certain specified diagnostic services
  ○ a therapy service
  ○ social work assistance
* all mental illness and mental handicap hospitals that were open in 1985 should be closed
* everyone over 85 should have a key worker
* referrals from GPs to specialist medical services should be reduced by 20%
* 40% of outpatient consultations with specialist medical staff should occur in locations other than District General Hospitals
* 80% of surgical interventions should be bloodless by 2002
* 60% of surgery should be day case by 2002
* hospital acute beds in DGHs should be reduced by at least 40% by 2002.'

(WHPF 1992, p. 9)

These benchmarks were used by the chief nursing offices of England, Wales, Scotland and Northern Ireland when they:

'invited a group of nursing leaders and other professional colleagues to consider these issues at a seminar at Heathrow.'

(DoH 1993, p. 1)

This group identified eight strategic issues for nursing and midwifery:
'• What will be the context in which nurses will work?
• What will be the contribution of nursing to meeting the needs of individuals?
• How will substitution impact on the role of nursing?
• How will the public react to the changed role of nursing?
• How will teamwork be developed with other carers in the health and social care spheres?
• How will professional accountability, authority and responsibility be altered?
• How will regulation impact on quality?
• What will be the implications for initial education and training, retraining and continuous training?'

(DoH 1993, p. 7)

These issues will now be used in this chapter as a framework to consider the question of health careers in the twenty-first century.

What will be the context in which nurses will work?

The Heathrow debate explored the wide-ranging changes occurring within the NHS, the future flexibility required of care givers whatever their position or background, and concluded this section with the following paragraph:

'Faced with changes of this magnitude there will be an urgent need for a new view of the role of nursing across the board. This will involve not only a reorientation towards a new equilibrium; it will also be necessary to consider how to prepare both existing and future nurses for an environment that is characterised by constant change. Change management is rarely simple, and seldom undertaken on this scale.'

(DoH 1994, para, 41, p. 8)

One view of the future has been given by the WHPF (1992) and most nurses, who have been thinking about the current changes and possible future scenarios, would endorse this thinking and approach. The shift to community rather than hospital care has already begun, although currently the resources are still trapped within the hospital sector. There are a great number of players involved: informal carers, the private and voluntary sector, GP fund-holders, social services and local authorities. How will nursing and midwifery interact with these players? Will this interaction be through a specific employer, or will nurses like doctors set up group practices to deliver nursing care? Moccia (1990) feels that nurses are ideally placed through working with individuals, families and communities to do the most to promote health and healing 'outside of our traditionally institution based delivery system' (p. 612). She goes on to say that this would be dependent on:

> 'redirecting the re-imbursement stream from public and provide payors away from tertiary care settings and making it available for providers other than physicians, such as nurse primary care providers, in community based settings such as home health care agencies and community nursing centers.'
>
> (Moccia 1990, p. 612)

Would this model fit with our present group of community nurses and health visitors? Is the context issue not only one of service delivery but also service delivery *by whom*? It may be that the changes necessary in nursing and health visiting to meet the new world needs will not be on such a grand scale as the changes necessary in other professional groups. Consider how doctors have brought 'new' players into the care provision field: physicians' assistants, surgeons' assistants, paramedics, probably all very able providers of care, but all totally responsible to doctors. Of course by the twenty-first century these new groups may be seeking recognition and independence from medicine!

Nurses do however, need to find a way of gaining political and economic recognition of their contribution to health gain. The focus of nursing and the contribution of nurses has been, and is, constantly changing. Experimental work by nurses in care areas is beginning to show the contribution to health that can be made (Pearson 1984; Kristjanson & Chalmers 1991). Salvage (1992) describes a new philosophy of nursing:

> 'The New Nursing began in the UK in the early 1970s, with the new departments of nursing in universities and polytechnics generating interest in nursing theory. They drew heavily on work from the USA, which sought to redefine the nurse's role in order to assert its unique contribution to healing (Henderson 1966), leading to claims for greater status, when the women's movement began to change assumptions about nurse's subordination to medicine. Meanwhile better standards of education, higher expectation and nascent consumerism provoked a reappraisal of the client/expert relationship on both sides of the Atlantic.'
>
> (Salvage 1992, p. 11)

It would seem that we are still struggling around these areas of concern. It seems that even when evidence is produced from research it is 'difficult' for general managers and other professions to acknowledge the contribution of nursing. An example of this is the research carried out at the Oxford Nursing Development Unit (ONDU) here in England. For a period of 15 months, elderly people were involved in a randomised controlled trial between the ONDU and a district general hospital. Salvage (1992) summarises the results:

'The results supported the hypotheses that patients transferred to the unit for therapeutic nursing received better and more consistent care than their district general hospital counterparts; became more independent; were more satisfied with their nursing; were generally as satisfied with life; had a shorter average stay in acute care; and incurred lower average costs. A surprise finding was a statistically significant reduction in the death rate of ONDU patients while in hospital, compared to the control group.'

(Salvage 1992, p. 16)

This work had shown that nurses could work in creative and innovative ways, that they had a contribution to make to health gain. Just how far this contribution could have gone is not clear:

'the ONDU inevitably had its share of problems, and the hostility of some doctors eventually led to its closure.'

(Salvage 1992, p. 17).

The second of the WHPF benchmarks is interesting mainly because it questions the contribution that could be made by nurses, midwives and health visitors in association with other professionals and practitioners. Could this be the beginning of polyclinics, nursing beds in a local setting, and a blurring of health and social professionals' contribution?

In every country there is consideration of the economic consequences of providing health care. In the United States there is real concern:

'there is a growing consensus that the nations' health care system is increasingly inadequate to meet the real health care needs of the population, that the public is increasingly dissatisfied with both the quality and cost of services, and that there will inevitably be a change in how the system is financed.

(Moccia 1990, p. 607)

There is another 'cost manager' emerging in the UK health scene, which has been present in the United States for some time and which has had a major controlling role in clinical decisions. This is the role played by the insurance companies who provide private insurance. Hillary Clinton (1995), recently described the current experience of women in the United States who, having given birth to their babies, are then threatened with separation from the baby because the insurance company would pay for *their* hospitalisation, but not for the babies'.

Anatole Kaletsky in *The Times*, posited an economic view of the NHS in July 1994, claiming that 'Britain's Health Service is by far the most efficient in the world':

> 'In fact, the NHS is so astonishingly efficient compared with America's privately financed and market-driven system that British taxpayers effectively get medical cover for everyone under 65 as a free bonus: our Government spends 5.5 per cent of GNP to cover everyone in the country, while in America it costs 5.9 per cent of GNP just to cover the old, poor and unemployed.'
>
> (Kaletsky 1994, p. 29)

Comparisons are being made all the time: How much? How many? What do we do with them? An understanding of the economic arguments is useful – we have less doctors per 1000 population than most other countries. Only the United States has less hospital beds than us. As these figures were based on OECD health data for 1993, we may now as a nation have considerably less beds. It would seem that all of us involved in delivering health care in the UK are pretty good at it, against considerable odds! However, Britain is not a rich country, in fact it has the second lowest standard of living in western Europe after Portugal (Ham & Cook 1995). This calculation refers to middle managers, so what must the outlook be for people who are unemployed or in less skilled jobs, or for single parents? Low standards of living must have an impact on health (Townsend & Davidson 1982; Townsend *et al.* 1988; Smith *et al.* 1990). So bearing all these factors in mind we move on.

What will be the contribution of nursing to meeting the needs of individuals?

This is an interesting question. Has there yet been a suggestion that nurses will stop meeting the needs of individuals? The Heathrow debate identified:

> 'Certain key tasks to be undertaken will include: careful, thoughtful needs assessment, using a technical framework but in a personal way; offering information, advice and comfort to patients and carers, while acknowledging their individual identities; and delivering effective care.'
>
> (DoH 1993, para. 48, p. 10)

The suggestion in the literature is that the contribution of nursing to meeting the needs of individuals, families and communities will get stronger and stronger:

'Powerful forces have radically changed the scope and complexity of health sciences and the delivery of health care. These forces will increase and alter the body of nursing knowledge, change the way health professionals practice, and modify the system of health care delivery. Recent advances in molecular and cell biology, immunology and microbiology have opened new avenues to preventive, diagnostic, and curative strategies. The caring strategies within nursing's domain provide us with astonishing power for maintaining health and managing with illness.'

(Abdellah 1990, p. 513)

Change in any organisation has the potential for destabilisation. The changes that are currently occurring in the NHS, as well as the changes in the nursing profession, have left nurses, midwives and health visitors at an impasse in relation to the people they are used to interacting with, and yet we are powerful. The whole world is changing for us, but then the same applies to other professional groups.

Perhaps one of the reasons that professional colleagues are feeling confused is that they have been brought up to have strong feelings of affiliation to the organisational ethos, i.e. the NHS. Perhaps in the future the strong feelings of affiliation will be to the nursing profession in general, and the individuals, families and communities who need care in a much stronger sense. Education will take place in higher education, the training element will be in a variety of care settings, not just the NHS. Where does one place one's allegiance then? This could be a difficult position for managers of service to find themselves in as there will be no traditional relationships to depend upon. These arrangements will put the 'local v. national' pay discussions into another dimension, and may mean that NHS Trust managers will more actively second and support learners in order to recruit them at the point of registration. An interesting thought!

The Patient's Charter Standard (NHSE 1994), on the named nurse, midwife and health visitor:

'a named qualified nurse, midwife or health visitor will be responsible for each patient's nursing or midwifery care'

(NHSE 1994, p. 3)

is an interesting standard. From reading the monitoring reports (NHSE 1994), it appears that tremendous benefits have accrued. Some discerning readers may question the reliability of some of the quoted benefits, but that apart, had organisations reached such a state of chaos and turbulence that emulation of the medical model of individualism was seen as the way forward? Nurses and midwives work co-operatively

(Uden *et al.* 1992), not only in professional teams, but also in partnership with patients, clients, families and communities. This is what we need to build upon, a strong supportive professional base, working in partnership (as equal partners) for the benefit of patients and clients. The exact contribution will depend on some of the factors discussed previously, and moreover, the strength of the profession in accommodating and affecting change.

How will substitution impact on the role of nursing?

'In reality, there is likely to be a reallocation of tasks between nurses and others, including other professionals. Nurses must be prepared to develop and change, drawing on the evidence of what is effective. In the past others have driven the research agenda, and so controlled the process of innovation and change. For the future, nurses must ensure that they too understand this process, so that research underpins a new clarity about what nurses can do best.'

(DoH 1993, para 65, p. 12)

Is *substitution* the right word to explain this? Does it lead readers to think of something lesser being put in place of the correct care deliverer? Perhaps instead we should be thinking about *organisational shift.* There are no new players in this field, we have always had a wide range of people involved in delivering care, from informal carers (who are total experts in the total one-to-one care they give to the person they care for), to experts who offer their expertise across a range of people in both a specific and general sense.

More and more the delivery of health care is dependent on informal carers. With an increasingly ageing population, and scarce resources in the national budget to support health interventions and health care, informal carers will be even more in demand. This is probably a good thing, in that the medicalisation of old age is not necessarily a model that society wants. What is wanted surely is support and understanding to continue day after day, night after night giving care to family members. A sense of balance, of life being in equilibrium, of other things being possible. Perhaps substitution in this scenario, is nursing substituting for the family, offering support and direction, respite care in nursing beds, arranging time for carers to be themselves, and to pick up their lives with friends, partners and families. If nurses do not offer direct care, then arranging for a substitute must be their role.

At the other end of the spectrum, are nurses substituting for doctors? In 1984, the International Council of Nurses (ICN) instigated a study to investigate the political and legal situation of nursing as a profession.

The aim was to develop an official position of the ICN to assist member associations in evaluating the developing regulatory systems for nursing (Styles 1985). van Maanen (1990) gives an example:

'... is the nurse's responsibility and accountability for medical procedures such as the distribution of intravenous cytostatics. Although professional regulation stipulates that such an invasive medical intervention be performed by physicians only, the clinical reality is different. There are still many nurses carrying out procedures for which they are not legally covered.'

(van Maanen 1990, p. 919)

This example was given to try to illustrate the complex arrangements between statutory regulation of professional activity and formal legislation in a country. At times there appears to be a tension. Perhaps this is a constant feature of change or transition here in the UK. The recent issues surrounding junior doctors' hours of work (DoH 1990) will have brought these concerns to the fore in many organisations. There is a difference, however, between advancing nursing practice and *substituting* for medicine.

Advancing nursing practice (ANP) requires a wholesale commitment to further education and training. There are colleagues who think that ANP is just allowing nurses to do tasks which previously were done by doctors when clearly this is not the case. In the United States, the American Nurses Association (ANA) has called for a health care system that:

'facilitates the utilisation of the most cost-effective providers and therapeutic options in the most appropriate settings.'

(ANA 1991)

This would mean putting the needs of the patient and/or client first and fitting the care to their needs rather then those of the prevailing system.

An example of this approach on both sides of the Atlantic is patient-focused care. A recent report on this topic (Hurst 1995) identifies that patient-focused care is designed to:

'... eliminate process steps and ease the administrative and co-ordination burden through limiting the number of staff involved with each patient.'

(Hurst 1995, p. 1)

This approach must be the one that nurses must grasp, linking this back to the WHPF (1992) benchmark 'everyone over 85 should have a key worker.'

At the M.D. Anderson Cancer Center in Houston, Texas, all five-year survivors of breast cancer are cared for by an advanced nurse practitioner; the nurse and patient/client decide if referral back to a doctor is necessary judging against agreed criteria. The nurse manages the continuing care of this group of women. So many opportunities, in so many settings. Is this substitution or is this nurses doing the sort of work that they are good at, and taking the initiative?

How will the public react to the changed role of nursing?

'In response to these challenges, nurses cannot rest on their laurels. They must monitor how attitudes are changing and consider the implications. Then, building on their existing skills, they must take an active role, moving out to educate the public in all its guises to broaden the understanding of the nature of nursing through other roles.'

(DoH 1993, para. 76, p. 14)

Nursing does not take place in a vacuum, the changed role of nursing will be seen against a backdrop of changing roles of other professions and institutions.

Health for All (HFA) by the year 2000 (WHO 1985) is a driving force internationally and has resulted in the publication of the *Health of the Nation* documents in England (DoH 1992). The concept of HFA has its basis in partnerships, and equal access to health and social care, within an appropriate governmental framework. The influence of HFA can be seen in the benchmarks developed by the WHPF (1992), and interestingly the first benchmark:

'by 2002, targets on smoking, physical exercise and weight are met'

is not a medical intervention, it is about health promotion, health education, health support. Its achievement will require a partnership between members of the public, professional groups and providers of social services.

It is interesting that the question 'How will the public react to the changed role of nursing?', is asked as a serious question. The public may have a view of changes affecting nursing against a bigger backcloth of NHS changes. There is an underlying philosophy, probably arising out of HFA, that the public are, or should be, involved in the changes affecting their health care provision. The changes that have affected the health service since the late 1980s have been both swift and efficient. These changes have been brought about in order to balance service performance of efficiency, effectiveness and acceptability against public expectations of rights, wants and needs (DoH 1993), a difficult balance to make. In most instances the public have not been involved in these changes, instead they have been imposed.

Interestingly, members of the public are questioning the health reforms. This challenging is usually at a level that individual members of the public can relate to. Richard Phillips (1995) describes the pathways of two people with spinal problems: one himself with backache; and his father with neck trouble. Mr Phillips junior is in a fund-holding practice. Within a week he was receiving treatment in the NHS and is now on the way to recovery. Mr Phillips senior, who is not in a GP fund-holding practice, has been told that he must wait between six to ten months to see a physiotherapist! The phrase 'two-tier system' (Phillips 1995, p. 19) appears three times in this small, two column article. This article is not about responding to nursing, but rather systems, management and underpinning philosophies. It questions issues of access, equity, effectiveness and efficiency. It highlights that people in the street are aware of service provision, that they have a view and will, where possible, take every opportunity to voice it. Nurses need to be aware of this emerging interest and anxiety. How to respond to it is something we should be giving considerable thought to and should be accorded proper respect: public opinion is not dead, and professionals need to maintain their critical awareness of it.

On the same page was a larger article on the deregulation of medicines, and the ease with which they can be purchased from pharmacies:

'Self-medication is popular with the government as it could help reduce the NHS drugs bill, running at around £3.6 billion a year. The drug industry is also in favour of the profit-boosting trend, as are pharmacists, who increasingly promote themselves as high street consultants.'

(Doyle 1995, p. 19)

For some people this is obviously a welcome development, they have special and particular knowledge about their personal health, and can make informed judgements. The article identified some 16 items recently released from prescription regulations, some of which seem sensible for one-off treatment of a condition, but the temptation must surely be to continue self-medication. When this freedom for self-medication is considered against the debate around allowing nurses to prescribe from a limited list, one wonders what sort of world we will be living in in the twenty-first century if the prevailing logic persists!

Health is a scarce resource (Smith *et al.* 1990), it is not even an equally distributed resource at birth (Barker 1991). It is often taken for granted by individuals until something happens which questions its stability or continuity. Health is affected by so many factors: poverty, nutrition, environment, education, employment; the contribution that nurses can make could be seen as minimal. But in the past nurses and midwives have made major contributions to health provision. Today that contribution continues. There is a strongly emerging view that the most successful contributions have their basis firmly in partnership with the public, which would make asking the question about the public's perspective on changes in nursing a valid and realistic one (Kristjanson & Chalmers 1991; WHO 1995).

How will teamwork be developed with other carers in the health and social care spheres?

'Once again the nurses must look for where they can properly take a lead, not settle into a secondary role. The public will soon recognise if the contribution is good, and will rightly complain if there is fragmentation. At present perhaps nurses too often cannot use their training to the full; the changes ahead create real opportunities to work with others to capitalise on their strengths.'

(DoH 1993, para. 84, p. 15)

An interesting area of discussion is emerging in the research literature, that of the different ways of thinking about doctors and nurses (Grundstein-Amado 1992; Uden *et al.* 1992). The work that is being done is in the area of ethical reasoning, and provides very useful food for thought, particularly in the area of practice. Do we want the nurses, midwives and health visitors of the future to think more like a doctor, or do we want doctors to think more like them? Or do we want an acknowledgement that because of our different training and education, we think in different ways? This diversity of thought is very useful in problem solving for the benefit of patients and clients.

The study by Uden *et al.* (1992) in Sweden, focused on ethically difficult care situations. A qualitative method was used to collect 23 registered nurses' and 9 physicians' stories. The two groups related different kinds of stories, and they seemed to use different kinds of ethical reasoning, (see Table 2.1). It was interpreted by the researcher that this was due to the fact that the two professions have different tasks to accomplish and are trained in disciplines with different foci. This will be an important consideration for the education and training of future advanced nurse practitioners. This is possibly another indication that where possible shared learning should take place. One of the easiest

Table 2.1 Themes in nurses' and physicians' stories about ethically difficult care situations (Uden *et al.*, 1992).

Nurses' stories	Physicians' stories
Retrospective	Prospective
Health and daily living	Disease
Experiential knowledge	Scientific knowledge
Closeness to patient	Distance
Patient autonomy	Paternalism
Quality of life	Preserving life
Pessimism	Optimism
Death with dignity	Survival
Powerlessness	Power
Being together with colleagues	Being isolated as an individual

places for this to happen is in the clinical setting with doctors and nurses working together to refine their skill base.

The benchmarks produced by the the WHPF sub-group (WHPF 1992) give tremendous opportunities for team working, and for contributing across other than traditional areas of work. Consider the marvellous opportunities for nurses who work with people with learning difficulties, their working partnerships with social workers, voluntary organisations, and families and communities.

Another interesting opportunity for teamwork is that of the Healthy Cities initiative of the WHO.

'The project focuses on action for health promotion at city level. It endeavours to place health high on the agenda of political decision-makers, key groups in the city and the population at large. It aims to develop feasible strategies for reorienting public health endeavours at city level and to make prevention and health promotion a highly visible and community-supported enterprise.'

(Kickbusch 1989, p. 77)

The scheme started with 11 participating cities; now there are over 300 initiatives in Europe, Australia, Canada, the United States and some countries in the developing world. There has been concern within the WHO that the original intent of Health for All by the year 2000, and subsequently the Healthy Cities project, has changed.

'Public health at city level, like WHO as a public health organisation, has become a medical rather than an interdisciplinary enterprise. The health for all strategy asks WHO and its constituents to reform and concentrate on health while reaching out to others for intersectoral action and participation.'

(Kickbusch 1989, pp. 77–8)

It seems strange that in a climate where so much is spoken of the health of the public, through strategies such as the Health for All by the year 2000 (WHO 1985) and the Health of the Nation (DoH 1992), that all the major organisational changes occurring in the UK are placing medicine firmly in the driving seat. This is despite the recurring challenges to medical dominance voiced elsewhere in the literature (see Part IV by Morton-Cooper) The government's research and development (R&D) agenda is an interesting example. All the very senior appointments to R&D both at the DoH/NHSE level and at the regional office (RO) level are doctors. The R&D agenda was supposed to be about research and its implementation across the NHS, it seems strange therefore to be making medical appointments to all the posts, rather that going for different skills and backgrounds that would have given a good mix across the country, and a good basis for a think tank on R&D issues.

It can be seen that the clinical R&D activity is important, and that it requires management and direction, but then so do a lot of other NHS R&D activities. There are anxieties amongst other employees in the NHS, and in the research community, that large pieces of activity ripe for research or development will not now be addressed. An interesting development from a nursing point of view is the work done by Dr Nicky Cullum (1994) at the UK Cochrane Centre in Oxford. The centre is working collaboratively on the international network to 'prepare and maintain systematic reviews of randomised controlled trials (RCTs) of the effect of health care', (Cullum 1994, p. 5). It would appear that there are a number of nursing research studies that use this method, and of course qualitative methods with these trials are not excluded.

How will professional accountability, authority and responsibility be altered?

> 'A good grounding through education and training – with each nurse able to manage resources, balance care and economy, act decisively and give clear direction to others – will be crucial for all areas.'
>
> (DoH 1993, para. 95, p. 16)

The people involved in the Heathrow debate (DoH 1993), felt that 'contracting [will] clarify expectations and accountability' (p. 15) and that this would in turn lead to clearer differentiation of roles through such things as the WHPF benchmarks, or other similar benchmarks, and increased individual responsibility for what the nurses do. This is interesting in that to date there has been little national involvement of nurses and midwives in the contracting process, and although there is a shift to define outcomes, at the present time most outcomes are still focused on medical outcomes. There will be a need to move forward fairly quickly in defining nursing outcomes if the suggestion outlined in the Heathrow debate (DoH 1993), of effectiveness and efficiency are to be achieved. These achievements are key agenda items, and nursing and midwifery need to be seen to be making a contribution.

The suggestions outlined in the above paper (DoH 1993) of greater visibility of nurses; and this greater involvement in contentious areas of care, such as genetic counselling and euthanasia as examples of areas of increased accountability, must move thinking on to authority, responsibility and autonomy. This then requires thought about where and how nursing is to be offered and delivered. The degree of difference from where we are now, to where we want to be, and where the people who pay the bills want nursing to be, could form the basis of a very interesting social debate, and are relevant to a much wider audience than the people who met at Heathrow. Consideration of these factors could produce additional tensions in the areas of litigation, regulation and the provision of care as a whole.

What is evident from the literature, and from current practices, is that nurses will become greater risk takers, they will be acting in a more autonomous manner in a very changed environment. This risk taking is not something that all nurses are comfortable with, and certainly other professional groups will, and do have, difficulty with the concept. Those expert practitioners who in the past phrased their words in such a way as to allow a junior doctor to begin to think of a line of action, will in the future make their own decisions, implement the action and evaluate the outcome. Is this not what all registered practitioners should be doing, and their employers expecting from them? The loop links back to sound education and training, professional and organisational support, and the ability and acceptance to say, 'I don't know, show me'.

'Once doctors qualify there is an implicit assumption that they are skilled in all of the tasks necessary for the diagnosis and treatment of patients under their care or that, if they are not, they will call for assistance as required. With nurses it is assumed that the skill is absent unless it has been taught and tested.'

(McKee & Lessof 1992, p. 66)

How will regulation impact on quality?

'Increasingly, it will not be enough just to be the right person, it will be more important to do the right thing.'

(DoH 1993, para. 104, p. 17)

This phrase sounds as though the ideas contained in it are issues for the future. They are not, in fact they have been around since the first Acts of Parliament establishing the register for nurses in 1919. Society has had expectations of one who calls themselves a registered nurse. With the title comes responsibility and accountability. The section taken from the Heathrow document (DoH 1993) uses the phrase 'to do the right thing', and this makes one think naturally of autonomy.

Responsibility and accountability are fairly well understood and explained in the literature, the framework provided by the UKCC *Code of Professional Conduct* (UKCC 1992a), *The Scope of Professional Practice* (UKCC 1992b), and *Standards for the Administration of Medicines* (UKCC 1992c), go some way to explaining these concepts, but autonomy is something that is talked about without always the same degree of understanding. Gillon (1985), describes autonomy as 'self rule':

> 'a capacity to think, decide, and to act on the basis of such thought and decision freely and independently and without, as it says in the British passport, let or hindrance.'
>
> (Gillon 1985, p. 60)

He also feels that it is important:

> 'in the sphere of action ... to distinguish between, on the one hand, freedom, liberty, license, or simply doing what one wants to do and, on the other hand, acting autonomously, which may also be doing what one wants to do but on the basis of thought or reasoning.'
>
> (Gillon 1985, p. 60)

He then goes on to discuss autonomy of *thought*, autonomy of *will* and autonomy of *action*. Gillon argues that autonomy is not a constant, 'it is a characteristic possessed by people in varying degrees'(Gillon 1985, p. 62). If we are to advance the contribution of nursing practice as a reality we need to build into the process of learning, the development of autonomy as outlined by Gillon. Not in order to reduce or constrain anyone else's autonomy, but rather to support and respect other individuals' autonomy and through that improve professional practice, and the contribution to care for patients and clients.

But how does this fit with quality? Taking quality in its widest interpretation, and not just the process application that sometimes seems to be the norm in the NHS, this will require greater application to outcome measures, and the necessary differentiation between inputs and throughputs. There are of course even greater opportunities for Europe to 'interfere' in the area of regulation. In the future there may be a European version of what a nurse is. Regulation will perhaps become more difficult when nurses are working in non-traditional settings. At present the NHS in part regulates professional activity here in the UK, but will this relationship be the same in the future with other employers? It is important here to differentiate between organisational regulation and professional regulation each of which have different objectives.

What will be the implications for initial education and training, retraining and continuous training?

'So a wide variety of instruments – education, training, retraining, experimentation and research – must be focused on a common objective: change within continuity. To ensure that this happens, and that nurses are released to take up their opportunities, there will need to be a common purpose shared by policy-makers at the highest level, commissioners and providers. Close liaison between these parties will be vital, together with a clear and satisfactory method of handling the budget for training and development.'

(DoH 1993, para. 112, p. 19)

There are a variety of possible scenarios in this context, it could be that by the twenty-first century all nurses and midwives will be graduates at point of registration. This will put them on the same academic footing as other professional groups in the health sector. It does not mean that they will necessarily cost more. It is important to understand that academic attainment does not necessarily mean greater financial rewards, particularly in the public sector. What it should lead to is a greater ability to think, reason, argue and negotiate for the benefit of patients and clients. It should give nurses the confidence apparent in other professional groups to argue from a professional standpoint for the worth of their contribution. For an organisation to get the best return on such an educational investment there will be a need to have a system which can meet need within a philosophy of life-long learning (Senge 1990).

There are anxieties being voiced about the output of the Project 2000 nurse preparation programmes here in the UK, where the 'students cannot do this, or that'. These students have had a broader based programme than their predecessors in order to prepare them to work in comfort in both the community or the acute sectors of care. Their programme of education begins by looking at and gaining an understanding of health per se. Their learning should be grounded in health, not like so many of their forbears, looking first at disease, and then only coming to 'health' as a concept, by virtue of additional education and experience. Students are being educated, they are being taught to question and challenge, they are being encouraged to discuss and explore issues with people who have first-hand experience of delivering care. This approach needs to be encouraged, to be facilitated by experienced, knowledgeable practitioners. Students in the present system should never be told 'You are not paid to think nurse, you are paid to do!' This was said to me as a student nurse, and could still be being said in some clinical areas today, although it is to be hoped not. The students of today are the professionals of the future. They need to be made to feel confident and strong, they also need to know that it is right to acknowledge what they do not know, and be helped to find out in a way that is intelligible and accessible to them rather than by patronage as in earlier years.

Nursing assistants who subsequently became health care assistants (HCAs) have had a long tradition of service in the NHS, and have filled the gap left by student nurses when the Project 2000 programmes were introduced. HCAs are an interesting adjustment to the workforce and as such evoke strong feelings in the profession. HCAs have a training pathway based on National Vocational Qualifications (NVQs). There was no professional involvement in these NVQ developments, from the beginning the professional bodies deliberately distanced themselves from them, feeling that they were not part of the professional agenda (Dickson & Cole 1987). This is a decision we may regret in the future. HCAs are part of the new approach to providing care, they work closely with nursing teams, they are part of those teams.

Any health organisation will be looking to get the maximum effort from their staff. The level of that contribution will vary according to the needs of the customers buying the service and the consumers utilising the service. The customers are not necessarily outside the organisation: if the services offered are for example, radiology services or laboratory services, they may be established as support services for the other directories within a Trust. As a principle no internal customer or consumer should be treated differently from external customers or consumers. The internal and external tensions need to be managed, as do the delivery of a quality service and management of resources. Already there is an education and training need, and professional issues have not yet been discussed. Chaston (1994) feels that:

> 'for a workforce to be willing and able to deliver service quality, management must ensure employees are capable of fulfilling their job role through activities such as creating effective teams, establishing supervisory controls and minimising the occurrence of role conflict.'
>
> (Chaston 1994, p. 388)

There will be a continuing need for education and training for all employees in managerial, professional and research areas. In some organisations at present there is no clear strategy for identifying education and training needs and as a result no real resources to allocate to meeting any needs that are identified. In many organisations there is now a process of individual performance review (IPR), where the individual's performance is reviewed against agreed objectives and criteria, by a line manager, and as a result of this interaction, personal education and training needs can be identified. At an organisational level a different more strategic approach needs to be taken.

Peter Senge, the author of *The Fifth Discipline* (1990), has some very interesting ideas about organisations as learning environments, and within that the ability of organisations (and people within them) to learn from experience. He quotes Draper Kauffman Jnr (1980), a systems-thinking writer:

'When a temporary oversupply of workers develops in a particular field, everyone talks about the big surplus and young people are steered away from the field. Within a few years, this creates a short-age, jobs go begging, and young people are frantically urged into the field – which creates a surplus. Obviously, the best time to start training for a job is when people have been talking about a surplus for several years and few others are entering it. That way, you finish your training just as the shortage develops.'

Perhaps that is what we should be doing in nursing, rather than reducing numbers of student nurses now, because we do not have jobs for nurses coming out of the education system. This would lead to clinical areas having sufficient staff to cover the work being done, and also support students in the clinical areas. This would also mean that staff in all areas of work could have regular opportunity for re-education and training, for refreshment and updating. Senge (1990) talks about personal mastery in his book, not meaning to be in any way dominant, he sees it as:

'the discipline of continually clarifying and deepening our personal vision, of focusing our energies, of developing patience, and of seeing reality objectively. As such, it is an essential cornerstone of the learning organisation – the learning organisation's spiritual founda-tion. An organisation's commitment to and capacity for learning can be no greater than that of its members.'

(Senge 1990, p. 7)

The argument is a circular one as theoretically an organisation which values its members and encourages their development is likely to be an organisation which will thrive and develop. People will want to work there, their contribution will be valued, they will *contribute*. Such a simple concept, but one so difficult to achieve in many organisations. In many organisations the budget for training and development is inadequate for meeting people's needs. Often because there is no systematic appraisal of need, it is mis-spent. In some organisations all of the training budget is spent on meeting the training needs of a small group of staff whose education and training is proscribed in legislation or national negotiated agreements, i.e. midwives, health visitors and doctors.

There needs to be a new approach to education and training, which is more clearly focused on the organisation and the people within it.

Conclusion

So, what about health careers in the twenty-first century? The issues are definitely complex, and there are so many of them. If nurses and their employers could act corporately in this, there are tremendous opportunities to be had and great gains to be made in terms of range of practice and opportunity to contribute at differing levels of care: preventive care, primary care and secondary care. But consider some of the issues, it is a case of all change, new approaches, new developments, new players, new partners in providing care. Both professionals and general management colleagues need to think about who will be delivering that care, one thing is for sure, it will not be as it was before.

The business of delivering health care is changing rapidly, there is a need for fast, responsive, flexible creative workers. This brings with it a need for debate, discussion and communication. There is a need to understand the political agendas, the resource issues, issues around inequality, allocation of resources, or in the new parlance, rationing. Professional groups have a major part to play in this new business.

References

Abdellah, F.G. (1990) Reflections on a recurring theme. *Nursing Clinics of North America*, **25**(3), 509–16.

ANA (1991) *Nursing's Agenda For Health Care Reform*. American Nurses Association, Kansas City, MO.

Barker, D.J.P. (1991) The foetal and infant origins of inequalities in health in Britain. *Journal of Public Health Medicine*, **13**(2), 64–8.

Chaston, I. (1994) Internal customer management and service gaps within the National Health Service. *International Journal of Nursing Studies*, **31**(4), 380–90.

Clinton, H. (1995) The cost of living is never too high. *Evening Standard*, 2 October, 12.

Cullum, N. (1994) The Cochrane Collaboration: Nursing Must Be Involved! *Nursing Development News*. King's Fund Centre. Issue 7. June 1994.

Davies, C. (1990) *The Collapse of the Conventional Career.* English National Board, London.

Davies, C. & Rosser, J. (1986). *Processes of Discrimination: A Study of Women Working in the NHS.* DHSS, HMSO, London.

Dickson, N. & Cole, A. (1987) Nurse's little helper. *Nursing Times,* **83**(10), 24–6.

DoH (1990) *Heads of Agreement. Ministerial Group on Junior Doctors' Hours.* Department of Health, London.

DoH (1992) *The Health of the Nation. A Strategy for Health in England.* HMSO, London.

DoH (1993) *The Challenges for Nursing and Midwifery in the 21st Century – A report of the 'Heathrow debate'.* Department of Health, London.

Donovan, M. (1990) What do we need to change about nursing? *Journal of Nursing Administration,* **20**(12), December.

Doyle, C. (1995) When patients play doctor. *Daily Telegraph,* 19 September, 19.

Edwards, B. (1993) *The National Health Service: A Manager's Tale 1946–1992.* The Nuffield Provincial Hospital Trust, London.

Gillon, R. (1985) *Philosophical Medical Ethics.* John Wiley & Sons, Chichester.

Grundstein-Amado, R. (1992) Differences in ethical decision-making processes among nurses and doctors. *Journal of Advanced Nursing,* **17**, 129–37.

Ham, P. & Cook, M. (1995) Britain's middle class the poor men of Europe. *The Sunday Times,* 17 September.

Handy, C. (1984) *The Future of Work.* Robinson, Oxford.

Handy, C. (1989) *The Age of Unreason.* Arrow Books, London.

Henderson, V. (1966) *The Nature of Nursing.* Collier Macmillan, London.

House of Commons (1984) *The First Report from the Social Services Committee: Session 1983–84. Griffiths NHS Management Inquiry Report.* HMSO, London.

Hurst, K. (1995) *Progress with Patient-focused Care in the United Kingdom.* National Health Service Executive, London.

Kaletsky, A. (1994) Prescribing markets as NHS servant not master. *The Times,* 29 July.

Kauffman, D. Jnr (1980) *Systems 1: An Introduction to Systems Thinking.* Future Systems Inc., Minneapolis, MN.

Kickbusch, I. (1989) Healthy cities: a working project and a growing movement. *Health Promotion,* **4**(2), 77–82.

Kristjanson, L.J. & Chalmers, K.I. (1991) Preventive work with families: issues facing public health nurses. *Journal of Advanced Nursing,* **16**, 147–53.

van Maanen, H.M.Th. (1990) Nursing in transition: an analysis of the state of the art in relation to the conditions of practice and societies expectations. *Journal of Advanced Nursing,* **15**, 914–24.

McKee, M. & Lessof, L. (1992) Nurse and doctor: whose task is it anyway? In: *Policy Issues in Nursing,* (eds J. Robinson, A. Gray & R. Elkan). Open University Press, Milton Keynes.

Mangan, P. (1994) The collapse of the conventional career. *Nursing Times,* **90**(16).

Moccia, P. (1990) Towards the future: how could 2 million Registered Nurses not be enough? *Nursing Clinics of North America,* **25**(3).

NHSE (1994) *The Patient's Charter: The Named Nurse, Midwife and Health Visitor – Checking that it Happens.* National Health Service Executive, London.

Pearson, A. (1984) The Burford experience. *Nursing Times,* **159**(22), 32–5.

Phillips, R. (1995) The two tiers of pain care. *Daily Telegraph.* 19 September, 19.

Robinson, J. (1992) Introduction: beginning the study of nursing policy. In: *Policy Issues in Nursing,* (eds J. Robinson, A. Gray & R. Elkan). Open University Press, Milton Keynes.

Robinson, K. (1992) The nursing workforce: aspect of inequality. In: *Policy Issues in Nursing,* (eds J. Robinson, A. Gray & R. Elkan). Open University Press, Milton Keynes.

RCN (1994) *Into the 90s: A Discussion Document on the Future of Health Visiting Practice.* Royal College of Nursing, London.

Salvage, J. (1992) New nursing: empowering patients or empowering nurses? In: *Policy Issues in Nursing,* (eds J. Robinson, A. Gray & R. Elkan). Open University Press, Milton Keynes.

Senge, P.M. (1990) *The Fifth Discipline: The Art and Practice of The Learning Organisation.* Century Business, London.

Smith, G.D., Bartley, M. & Blane, D. (1990) The Black report on socio-economic inequalities in health 10 years on. *British Medical Journal,* **301**, 18–25 August, 373–7.

Styles, M.M. (1985) *Project on the Regulation of Nursing. International Council of Nurses,* Geneva.

Townsend, P. & Davidson, N. (1982) *Inequalities in Health: the Black Report.* Harmondsworth, London.

Townsend, P., Davidson, N. & Whitehead, M. (1988) *Inequalities in Health: The Black Report and the Health Divide.* Harmondsworth, London.

Uden, G., Norberg, A., Lindseth, A. & Marhaug, V. (1992) Ethical reasoning in nurses' and physicians' stories about care episodes. *Journal of Advanced Nursing,* **17**, 1028–34.

UKCC (1992a) *Code of Professional Conduct.* United Kingdom Central Council for Nursing, Midwifery and Health Visiting, London.

UKCC (1992b) *The Scope of Professional Practice.* United Kingdom Central Council for Nursing, Midwifery and Health Visiting, London.

UKCC (1992c) *Standards for the Administration of Medicines.* United Kingdom Central Council for Nursing, Midwifery and Health Visiting, London.

WHO (1985). *Targets for Health for All. Targets in Support of the European Regional Strategy for Health for All.* World Health Organization, Copenhagen.

WHO (1995) *Nurses Work to Narrow the Health Divide.* Press release EURO/03/95. World Health Organization, Copenhagen.

WHPF (1992) *Health and Social Care 2010: A Program of Work for Services.* Welsh Health Planning Forum subgroup, Cardiff.

Witz, A. (1994) The challenge of nursing. In: *Challenging Medicine,* (eds J. Gabe, D. Kelleher & G. Williams). Routledge, London.

3
Dimensions of Organisational Health

Margaret Bamford and
Alison Morton-Cooper

The concept of occupational health is a well-established feature of the health and health management literature internationally. This chapter takes a further conceptual leap into the problematic area of health in organisations by bringing together, possibly for the first time, the more holistic perspective of organisational health. *From this broader perspective the physiological, psychological and psychosocial aspects of health are considered pragmatically from the positions of both employer and employee. What priorities should a manager place on organisational health, and what indices can be used to assess the health status of an organisation and its employees?*

The authors argue that the previous narrow (and often marginalised) perspective of occupational health has at times disenfranchised people within organisations, by relegating health issues to the domain of specialist professionals. In the interests of greater health democracy they suggest that more attention should be paid to organisational conceptualisations of health, in the firm belief that this will actually help to clarify the health demands of day-to-day working, putting managers and employees in a better strategic and personal position to manage health issues more effectively.

Issues such as changing work and shift patterns, assessment of the quality of working life and the management of emotional as well as physical health in the workplace are the central features of this chapter.

Introduction

Work gives people place and position in society; it gives them the potential to earn money, to keep themselves and their families. It is seen as a 'good' thing to have by most people.

Work continues to play a central role in the lives of people in the UK. The study of that relationship has exercised many disciplines, psychologists, sociologists, health professionals, ergonomists and of course, students of management. Work takes place within organisations, some of which are more formal than others. A term which is commonly used to describe this area of study, particularly from a management perspective, is organisational behaviour (OB).

It could be argued that OB and organisational health (OH) are the same thing. However, OB refers to topics such as:

'work attendance, motivation, commitment, obedience, productivity, leadership, team work and overcoming resistance to change, ... [rather than] issues of ethics, corporate responsibility, identity, power and conflict, exploitation, personal autonomy, greed, obsession and violence.'

(Corbett 1994, p.3)

Organisational health on the other hand provides an opportunity to consider the symbiotic relationship between organisations and the people working within them. Corbett (1994) goes on to state:

'work organisations can be understood not only as environments in which people produce work, but also as places where work produces people. Hence, any discussion of what people want or need out of work (particularly paid employment) cannot be isolated from the context of that work environment.'

(Corbett 1994, p. 9)

The whole process of looking at work, the environment in which it takes place and the consequences is complex, complicated and multi-factorial. It is interesting that when speaking to people about organisational health, they have turned this around and instead used the phrase 'oh, yes, a sick organisation'. Do we recognise sickness and illness in an organisation better than health? We certainly know about 'sick buildings':

'Sick Building Syndrome (SBS) is used to describe a higher than expected incidence of symptoms such as irritation of the eye, nose and throat, headaches, nausea, and mental fatigue. There appears to be no single overriding cause of SBS, which tends to occur more frequently in buildings that are well sealed and air conditioned or mechanically ventilated. Various contributory factors have been associated with SBS, including inadequate ventilation, thermal discomfort, low humidity, air pollution, as well as such factors as low morale and dissatisfaction with working conditions.'

(Health and Safety Commission (HSC) 1991, p. 41)

There are many hazards which could affect a worker from a psychological and/or social point of view, but which stem from the organisation rather than what the person brings to work with them. Examples would include working unsociable hours, abuse at work, feelings of stress, lack of control in work processes, and problems associated with shift working or employee boredom.

There are physical stressors in the workplace which can affect a person psychosocially, e.g. poor visibility and eye strain, excessive noise, vibration, heat, cold, humidity, wind, motion, perceived dangers such as work overload or underload, pressures of shiftwork and combinations of these (Poulton 1978). Blaxter (1990) identifies psychosocial health as one of the four dimensions of health, the other three being unfitness or fitness, disease and impairment or their absence, and experienced illness or freedom from illness.

It is important for people at work to be considered holistically, and for there to be an acknowledgement that their health can be adversely affected by the work that they do. Equally well, factors affecting their psychosocial health away from work can have an effect on work performance, i.e. divorce, separation, bereavement, moving house, changing job. It is also vital to consider the nature and social context of the work environment (Heerwagan *et al.* 1995) and the behaviour and social expectations of the people with whom they are expected to work (Spurgeon & Barwell 1995; Turnbull 1995).

When considering the history of work in society, it is important to remember time and context. The Greeks and Romans had slaves to do their work, whilst the Hebrews felt that they gained spiritual dignity through the enactment of work. The early Christians believed that work made one healthy; it was a useful diversion from the threat of sinful thoughts, habits and other diversions. Work was also seen (particularly for the erring lower classes) as a penance for their inopportune fall from Grace. The Protestant Christians who followed the teaching of Luther saw work as a way of serving God. But where does this leave the average employee today?

There is considerable debate regarding the future of work; the type of work it will be, how it will be carried out, where it will be done and who will do it (Toffler 1980; Handy 1989). Handy raises the notion of wage work, fee work, gift work and study work. This is a difficult cognitive transition for many people who have perhaps been raised on the Protestant work ethic to make, and requires a different way of thinking about work. It may mean that people will need to be paid more for the smaller proportion of formal, i.e. wage work that they do.

Harpaz (1989) discusses instrumental (economic) reasons for work, and non-instrumental reasons which he describes as 'expressive in nature'. He cites the term used by Warr (1982), 'non-financial employment commitment' (Harpaz 1989, p. 147) Harpaz explored this concept internationally, asking whether people would continue to work if they won a lottery or inherited so much money that they would no longer have any financial incentive. From a sample of 840, 68.8% of men and women in the UK said that they would continue to work. However, as this was only an hypothetical question, no one knows what would happen in reality?

Changes in organisational structure

Improvements in the current working environment are barely credible compared to conditions of even 20–30 years ago. Our knowledge and understanding of the effects of poor working conditions and environments have increased in tandem. Since the mid-1980s in particular, there has been a dramatic change in the range and type of work organisations in the UK and across the globe with the rise of sophisticated communication technologies and the increased viability of home working. In health care, some organisations have found themselves reorganised or abolished altogether, with the attendant proliferation of private and independent sector organisations and the evolution of new and emerging organisations such as (in the UK) GP fund-holders. Some organisations have restructured, reconfigured or redefined their roles, examples being those of acute and community sector NHS (National Health Service) Trusts and health commissioners, all of which have been charged with seeking new and more cost-effective ways of moving health care forward (Ferlie *et al.* 1994).

Although some organisations still remain which could be described as bureaucratic and rational, many of the new or emerging health organisations are quite different. These organisations have evolved from the NHS and Community Care Act 1990, which itself flowed from the government white paper, *Working for Patients* (DoH 1989). Structures may have changed, but they tend to be less hierarchical, are flatter in design, and in some instances they represent less formal and traditional ways of working in their search for new ways of increasing productivity and flexibility (Ferlie & Pettigrew 1996).

People and work in organisations

In a recent study (Bamford 1993) of employees' perceptions of their health carried out in the West Midlands (UK), and covering 14 different large organisations (see Table 3.1), it was found that 58 people (13%) felt

Table 3.1   Research population information.

	Number of people
Gender responses	
Male	290 (63%)
Female	165 (36%)
Age	
16–24	43 (9%)
25–34	99 (22%)
35–44	140 (31%)
45–54	117 (25%)
55–64	52 (11%)
Type of organisation surveyed: returned questionnaire ($n = 70$)	
An emergency service	41 (59%)
Metal components factory	45 (64%)
A tyre maker	20 (29%)
Car components manufacturer	36 (51%)
NHS Trust	36 (51%)
Local Education Authority	34 (48%)
Local Authority Property services	37 (53%)
A university	32 (46%)
An electrical components factory	28 (40%)
A porcelain manufacturer	40 (57%)
A metal components factory	25 (36%)
A chemical manufacturer	21 (30%)
An electrical company	50 (71%)
A catering company ($n = 40$)	13 (33%)

their health had been affected for good by the work they did; 94 people (20%) felt their health had been affected fairly by the work that they did; 126 (27%) felt there had been no effect; 124 (27%) felt the effect had been poor and 31 (7%) felt the effect had been bad (see Table 3.2). Twenty-six people (6%) did not respond to this question, this out of a total of 459 returned questionnaires (48% response rate).

When looking at the different aspects of the scale, a third of the sample

Table 3.2

Effect	Number of people
Good (Group 1)	58 (13%)
Fair (Group 2)	94 (20%)
No effect (Group 3)	126 (27%)
Poor (Group 4)	124 (27%)
Bad (Group 5)	31 (7%)
No response	26 (6%)
Total	459 (100%)

(152) felt that work had been positive in relationship to their health, scoring good or fair, (33%). This figure did not change dramatically when divided for the sexes (males 33% and females 34%).

For the 'no effect' category the overall figure of 126 (27%) for both sexes was recorded, and again there were no significant differences when broken down into the sexes (males 27% and females 28%).

In the 'poor' effect category an overall response rate of 124 (27%) was recorded for both sexes. This did not vary greatly when divided for the sexes (males 28% and females 25%). In the 'bad' category there was a general response of 31 (7%) for both sexes and again no significant difference was found when divided for the sexes (males 6% and females 7%). However, if the two negative comment groups, 4 and 5, are taken together, they total 155 (34%), the same percentage as for the positive group.

The comments that people made to support their perception of the effects of work on health are as follows:

- Group 1.   Positive comments associated with 'good' scores were:

  o 'If I've done my job properly, it makes me feel good, and I feel good most of the time.
  o 'I love my work, and it provides me with fulfilment.'

- Group 2.   In the group who recorded 'fair' to this question, some of the comments made were less positive than would be expected from the numerical score, for example:

  o 'Worry and travelling, especially driving at speed.'
  o 'Enjoyable job, some drawbacks with over commitment to research interests and consequent stress.'
  o 'Sometimes in my job it can become stressful and worrying.'

  These people seem to see fair as meaning 'only fair'. Other people in this group made more positive comments:

  o 'It is hard work, but I enjoy it and if I am away from it for more than a week, I tend to become despondent.'
  o 'I enjoy my employment, and never regretted enrolling into my occupation.'

- Group 3.   In the group of people who felt that work had had 'no effect' on their health, there were a large number of 'no comments'; however, comments that were made included:

  o 'Physical aspects are good for you, but shifts and smoke inhalation are bad for you.'
  o 'Despite having worked in a foundry during my early working life, I

seem to have been fortunate enough to have escaped the respiratory complaints which used to prevail in this industry. Subsequent employment has been in relatively non-hazardous environments.'

○ 'Health not really affected although the last nine years at work has personally been depressing as I do not really enjoy my present job. I find it difficult to get out of my present job situation.'

○ 'Shift work and piece work are not ideal working conditions but they don't seem to have any effect on me.'

In this group the responses seem to be both positive and negative. There does seem to be an understanding of the effects of work on health and how that affects individuals.

- Group 4. Of the people who scored 4 or 'poor' to this question, the following comments were recorded:

  ○ 'I am stressed and unhappy, unfulfilled and angered by the leadership of the management.'

  ○ 'Not being able to move from your seat, 10 minute break in morning, 20 minutes for lunch and 10 minutes of an afternoon is insufficient for an 8 hour day.'

  ○ 'Eyesight impaired by constant close work.'

  ○ 'Progressive deafness over 40 years in noise.'

  ○ 'Hearing loss, due to noise levels. Back ache due to bending and lifting.'

  ○ 'Ladder climbing, installation, work pressure brings on angina pains in my chest.'

Out of this group of 124 people, 50 people included 'stress' or 'pressure' in their answer. Comments from 28 men (34%) included:

○ 'Stress levels can be high.'

○ 'Smoke inhalation and intense short periods of stress.'

Comments from 22 women (52%) included:

○ 'Too much stress, too many demands.'

○ 'At various times/jobs, self-perception/stress/confidence in future are all job related, and reflect current stability of and satisfaction with job.'

○ 'On the whole my job is satisfying, however, there is a certain amount of stress, the usual effect is weight loss (good or bad?).'

People have a mixed perception of health in relation to work, some aspects are purely physical, others perceived more as psychological.

- Group 5.   In the group who felt that work had had a 'bad' effect on their health, the following comments were recorded:

  o 'A lot of mental stress working for present employer, due to it setting people on, then making them redundant.'
  o 'Due to the emergency nature of my work sometimes adequate precautions against injury, long or short term, emotional and physical, can not be taken.'
  o 'Excessive strain from short staffing and further study ... raised blood pressure has been a symptom of stress.'

Other people quoted specific physical effects: tenosynovitis, previous injuries, backache, eye strain, reduced hearing; all these conditions related to occupation in the opinion of the respondents.

People have mixed views about the effect of the work and health interface, some view events positively, others negatively, some have not thought about the issue at all. Loscocco and Roschelle (1991), in their review of the literature on influences on the quality of work and non-work life, have focused very much on what they see as the most common assessment in this area which is individual attitudes. They feel that people's past and projected work experiences affect their reactions to jobs. This would be an important factor when considering organisational health as there is a great need to consider people as individuals. Spurgeon and Barwell (1995) would take this argument at little further:

'Physical and emotional deprivation in childhood, poor parental models and low self-esteem can all act as early agents that make people more vulnerable to work adjustment in later life.'

(Spurgeon & Barwell 1995, p. 109)

What constitutes organisational health?

Bruhn and Chesney (1994) feel that the concept of a healthy organisation is idealistic. They feel that:

'Organisations are living systems with their own needs and life cycles. Like other living things, they experience change and conflict as they grow and develop.'

(Bruhn & Chesney 1994 p. 21)

This is an interesting analogy to make. Most organisations are the sum of the parts that constitute them. In most instances these parts are the people in the organisation. Organisations will never remain static, some will go through major change and reorganisations. Others will adjust at the margins which is what happened within the NHS during the early reorganisations of the 1980s.

The same type of major change can be seen in other areas of the public sector: energy, transport, housing and education. The organisations providing these 'services' are now functioning totally differently to their performance of even 10 years ago. For one thing some of them would now be considered to be in the private rather than the public sector. Market forces are prevailing. This is a difficult concept for the average person to come to terms with. Services which were considered to be 'of the public good' are being sold off, acquiring shareholders and are expected to return both a service *and* a profit. The breadth and range of change in organisations can cause feelings of anxiety for the people working in them and for those citizens who depend on the services they provide.

Indices of organisational health and diagnostic tools

What constitutes a healthy organisation? Bruhn and Chesney (1994) see the characteristics of a healthy organisation as being composed of three major elements: the organisational culture, leadership issues, and employees. (see Fig. 3.1) Their perspective is very much from an organisational view, and acknowledges that organisations, in addition to being sick themselves, can through their behaviour cause individuals to experience ill-health and sickness.

Williams (1994) in his exploration of ideas for creating healthy work organisations identifies four areas for consideration: environmental factors, physical health, mental (psychological) health and social health. He relates these four areas to internal and external factors, but is very focused on the person, occupational health and safety aspects, with little mention of 'managerial' factors in influencing an organisation's health.

Quality of working life (QWL)

QWL is seen by Kerce and Booth-Kewley (1993, p. 189) as 'a way of thinking about people, work and organisations':

> 'a group of methods or technologies for making the work environment more productive and more satisfying to workers. These methods are distinguished from other productively or organisational developmental efforts in that their focus is on outcomes for the employee rather than for management.'
>
> (Kerce & Booth-Kewley 1993, p. 190)

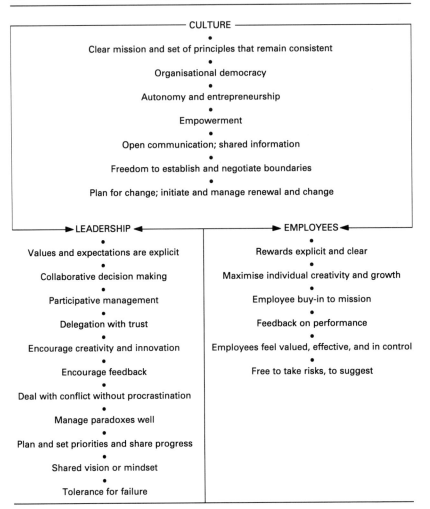

Fig. 3.1 Characteristics of healthy organisations. Reproduced with permission from Bruhn, J.G. & Chesney, A.P. (1994) Diagnosing the health of organizations, *Health Care Supervision*, **13**(2), Fig. 1, p. 25, © 1994, Aspen Publishers, Inc.

This focus on outcomes for employees rather than management is an interesting notion. The whole focus of organisations and managers should be to maximise the contribution and therefore the productivity of employees.

Kerce and Booth-Kewley found from their survey of the literature that there has been a change in perceptions of positive QWL environment. Previously such an environment would have been described as one providing factors such as: stability of employment, adequate income, benefits, fair treatment, due process, and a safe and secure place to work (Mirvis & Lawler 1984, cited in Kerce & Booth-Kewley 1993). But times are changing and a broader definition is needed to express what is understood by QWL by current workers. A positive QWL environment should now include:

'job challenge commensurate with individual's level of education, autonomy, responsibility, good co-worker relationships, good supervision and the opportunity to develop individual interests and abilities.'

(Kerce & Booth-Kewley 1993, p. 190–91)

These characteristics will be familiar to many people employed in the health care sector, as either their personal experience of work or the characteristics they aspire to attain in their own work place. Kerce and Booth-Kewley (1993) assert that many organisations do not acknowledge these changing attitudes and perceptions, and have not been responsive in either their re-structuring of work or their reward strategies.

It is important to remember cultural factors. Behaviour that would be acceptable and 'normal' in the UK may not be acceptable in other countries. Other countries and cultures will have different needs, values and standards. It is important for managers and other employees to take these factors into account when employing or working with people from different societies; there may be implications for risk taking and for leadership behaviour.

Efraty and Sirgy (1990) in looking at the effects of QWL on employee's behavioural responses, surveyed eight organisations providing care to the elderly in a large city in the American Midwest. Three organisations provided services in nursing homes and five in the community. The researchers explored four areas of concern which were drawn from Maslow's hierarchy of need (1954) and modified. The four categories were: survival needs, which included factors such as security needs and pay; social needs, examples including interpersonal interactions, friendship, needs for membership and 'being-in-the-know in a significant social group'; ego needs, needs of self-esteem and autonomy; and self-actualisation needs. The results identified that:

'... the more employees satisfy survival, social, ego and self-actualization needs in the organisation, the more they will be identified with the organisation, the more they will derive satisfaction from their/his job [sic], the more involved they will be in their/his job, the more they will exert effort in their job, and the more effective they would be perceived by their/his superiors, and the less personal alienation they will experience.'

(Efraty & Sirgy 1990, p. 43–4)

These authors feel that there are messages for both managers and public policy makers in their work. They believe that energy should be put into enhancing the QWL of employees to meet the four categories of need identified. They feel that enhancing the QWL of employees will provide additional benefits to society as a whole by 'decreasing personal alienation, and therefore enriching people's lives with positive experiences.' (Efraty & Sirgy 1990, p. 44). But is this what work is seen to be about in the present climate of international competitiveness? Have we developed such a style that people are not considered to any great extent, as organisations retract, re-focus, reorganize? Is the energy going into keeping the organisation alive at all costs, to the detriment of the people working within it?

It is quite clear that what is happening in organisations, both to the organisations and the people working in them, are multi-factoral issues. It is no longer appropriate to be researching single factor issues, and wherever possible there should be integration to take account of a range of variables. Working life is not a collection of boxes, and events and people do not fit nicely into them. Workplaces are part of the community in which they are based and which they serve. They need to be seen as part of the public health. The public are at work in our workplaces; we should extend our thinking to include them in all health planning and provision that is going on in a community (WHO 1985; Bamford 1996).

The emotional health of organisations

Emotions, it would seem, are not welcome in the *rational* organisation. Employees may exhibit emotions (infrequently, and then only if they *must*), whilst managers are expected to remain immune to them, steadfastly retaining their (presumed?) natural objectivity and logic in the face of any *irrational* emotional forces. This 'gendering of emotion' perpetuates a tradition which couples emotion with women in direct opposition to reason and men: 'the consequences of this is that the former is denigrated in contrast with the latter, as is prevalent in male-stream [sic] scientific discourse' (Swan 1994, p. 91).

Emotions have the reputation of being chaotic, subjective and weak in the face of the bureaucratic preference for a rational base. Emotion is therefore marginalised in organisations, in the widely held belief that 'rationality and the control of organisations are not only inseparable but also necessary for effective organisational life' (Putnam & Mumby 1993).

The dominant assumption in Western psychology has been that emotions are simple disturbances of the efficient functioning of goal-directed behaviour, the implication being that emotion therefore interferes with our effective functioning, *getting in the way of* otherwise rational and decisive actions. This view is now being challenged, however, so that emotions may be understood:

> 'not to distort [our] rationality, but rather, the opposite: in the perturbations of the smooth surface of habit, of plans, of schemes that do not always go as we might have planned, we can sometimes catch a glimpse of something real in us that may point beyond the issue of our achieving our next goal.'

> (Oatley 1992, p. 410)

At the level of organisation there is yet another dimension, that of the *psychic prison*, an idea first explored in Plato's *Republic*, but related to modernity by the management writer Gareth Morgan. Morgan suggests that, like the people within the underground grave cited in Socrates' allegory, employees may become imprisoned or confined by the images, ideas, thoughts and actions to which conscious and unconscious social processes give rise. People can become 'trapped by favored [sic] ways of thinking', and by 'constructions of reality which at best give an imperfect grasp on the world'. While organisations may therefore be viewed as socially constructed realities, 'these constructions are often attributed an existence and power of their own that allow them to exercise a measure of control over their creators' (Morgan 1986, p. 199).

Morgan uses this idea to explain why some people resist change more readily than others, arguing that they are often the victims of their own misapprehensions. He examines organisations from the psychoanalytical perspective of repression, and from the feminist perspective of patriarchy, seeming to intimate that we are all at risk of falling prey to the blinding irrationalities of human feeling by failing to control our human impulses.

In his view, 'hidden forces' which lead us to over-depend on hierarchies and organisational rules can get in the way of being creative, organic and innovative. This bureaucratic emphasis on maintaining control (e.g. in standardisation procedures, benchmarking, scientific management) is therefore part of the human drive to maintain social and collective order in our lives:

> 'And in doing so, we create the myth that we are actually in control, and that we are more powerful than we really are. Much of the knowledge through which we organize our world can thus be seen as protecting us from the idea that, ultimately, we probably understand and control very little. Arrogance often hides weakness, and the idea that human beings, so small, puny and transient, can organize and

boast mastery of nature, is in many respects, a sign of [our] own vulnerability.'

(Morgan 1986, p. 214)

Thus our metaphorical drawbridges and lines of defence are drawn, so that perceived threat may be met with the time-honoured response: a negation of our human frailty and the paradoxical expression of our human strength. This entails on the one hand the expectation that we should be able and ready to confront and deal with our human problems, while on the other we have only meagre emotional resources on which to draw in times of need or trouble. It is interesting to note that employee resistance remains a persistent, significant and remarkable feature of contemporary organisations, and that throughout the twentieth century it has been the primary analytical concern of scholars of organisation as well as a pervasive feature of labour process practices (Collinson 1994, p. 25–6).

Fear of emotions

Psychotherapist and writer, Susie Orbach, is unequivocal about the problems people experience generally in expressing and coming to terms with their emotions in everyday life. She believes that we need to challenge our culturally transmitted fear of emotions, as this only exploits and distorts people's longings and desires:

'A fear of emotions curtails our health, our marriages, our relation-ships with children as well as our capacity for citizenship. Until we challenge the consensus that keeps us emotionally illiterate, our desire for recognition, for intimacy, for selfhood and for community will continue to appear in fragmented, distorted forms.'

(Orbach 1994, p. 6)

This phenomenon of *emotional illiteracy* is not new in the literature. John Macmurray, the Scottish Communitarian philosopher whose work is currently enjoying a renaissance in contemporary political circles, had very definite ideas on the subject in 1935. He lamented the human failure 'to educate the emotional life', arguing (somewhat emotionally!) that the exclusive concentration of training for the intellect, and the subse-quently relegation of the emotional life to a subordinate status could only make us 'capable of determining the means to human life and very little of living it'. The intellect, in Macmurray's opinion, arises directly from the emotional life. Emotion is therefore *the* unifying factor in life, so that:

'[A]ny education which is fully conscious of its functions must refuse to treat human life as a means to an end. It must insist that its sole duty is to develop the inherent capacity for a full human life. All true education is an education in living...'

(Macmurray 1935, p. 42–3)

It could be argued that this quest for emotional literacy has been popularised in the media generally in recent years by what has become the established 'stress' discourse. The concept of stress is certainly no stranger to health care staff, and to nurses and doctors particularly, (see, for example, Holland, 1994; Sutherland & Cooper, 1990). Nursing is 'generally acknowledged to be a stressful occupation in a stress filled society' (Jacobson & McGrath, 1983, p. xi), and there is little evidence to suggest that other health professionals fare any differently.

Problems of the stress discourse

The cost to the UK economy in terms of NHS treatment for stress-related disorders has been estimated at £5 billion a year, with the additional burdens of associated sickness benefits, early retirement or compensation payments and the cost of replacing staff falling heavily on employers and government alike (Meusz 1995, p. 1). The stress industry is manifested in the popular press and in the wealth of articles and self-help materials on offer for dealing with the phenomenon on a personal as well as organisational level.

The popularity of the stress concept is said to be due largely to research on life change events and illness, to the point that it has been described as the stress revolution (e.g. Smith 1993). It has elsewhere been claimed that the stress discourse has allowed for:

'a relatively straightforward and easy mass production of books, articles and PhDs, [so that stress] has gained legitimacy within and beyond academe on the basis of a seemingly objective and scientific method.'

(Newton *et al.* 1995, p. 48)

Newton *et al.* have warned that it is important to relate stress to other discourses, or there is a distinct danger of being seduced into believing that popular representations of stress constitute its reality. The difficulty with stress is that its power as a discourse lies in our not knowing whether we have become more stressed than before, so that stress surveys may just be measuring the power of (and therefore our engagement with) the stress discourse, rather than the real experience of stress.

Stress itself may therefore be caught up in the debate about work, so that in previous centuries it was perceived differently, either as honest hard work (characteristic of the Protestant work ethic), or as a service to a higher authority, as in early Christian and medieval conceptions of work and the notion of earning our due rewards in the after-life (see Ransome 1996, p. 99). The real power of stress lies in its linguistic usage, so that seen from a traditional Marxist perspective:

> '[S]tress, with its emphasis on individualism, apoliticism, ahistoriscism and so on can be seen as just one further reflection of a pervasive ideology which glosses over the inequalities of power reflected in existing social structures, and lays the blame primarily on the individual... People believe in the language of stress ... because they have swallowed capitalist ideology.'
>
> (Newton *et al.* 1995, p. 11)

It could be argued, however, that it is the more recent politicisation of stress which pervades the popular press and the management literature, so that occupational stress has been brought to the front-line of industrial relations. The modern expectation of all workers (across the organisational hierarchy) is the required ability to manage a fair share of the stress manufactured by the drive for corporate efficiency. Productivity, change in employment levels, and profitability are among the measures currently used to assess effectiveness within the UK public sector (Flanagan & Spurgeon 1996, p. 40), although they could also be described as the means advocated by central government for acquiring and maintaining economic 'competitiveness' generally (Board of Trade 1996).

Safeguarding emotional health in organisations

Strategies for identifying and managing job-related stress are a common feature of the management literature (e.g. Flannery 1990), with the emphasis focusing less on structural causes and more closely on the affected individual taking personal responsibility for creating and maintaining an assertive and balanced lifestyle based on emotional and physical 'fitness for purpose'. On the evidence currently available, it would seem reasonable to assert that human stress has been problematised and commodified, so that the responsibility people feel for 'taking control' of their lives may be part of an all-embracing political strategy to maintain control over populations.

For example, theories which ostensibly address the human difficulties experienced as the perceived consequence of stress, have relied heavily on the biological concept of adaptation, defined as 'the action or process of adapting to or modifying as to suit new conditions' (*Shorter Oxford English Dictionary*). Thus, the qualitative emphasis is placed on the 'person–environment fit', the onus being on the person – rather than the environment – to alter and adapt to suit prevailing or anticipated conditions. If stress really is the product of social and behavioural science research as Pollock has claimed (Pollock 1988, quoted in Newton *et al.* 1995), then this may be an example of what the sociologist Weber described as the iron cage of rationality; which is the end result of our attempts to enforce order on society by constantly measuring and quantifying our responses to human situations.

It is nevertheless a truism that stress is an important construct when considering the emotional impact of modern living. For most of us, stress may be a helpful way of describing the pressures and constraints inflicted on us by contemporary ways of working.

As such, popular conceptions of stress and its management have important implications for the maintenance of our psychological health in the workplace. It therefore deserves to be taken seriously as an organisational health issue, and accorded the proper respect as part of the wider psychological contract which exists between employer and employee (see Makin *et al.* 1996 for a full and frank discussion on the psychological elements of the economic contract).

Impact of occupational stress

Willcox (1994) describes occupational stress as:

'...a negatively perceived quality which as a result of inadequate coping with sources of stress, has negative mental and physical ill health consequences.'

(Willcox 1994, p. 54)

Many people at work will seek a medical opinion to support their feelings of illness, indeed many of them may need expert medical help. Until fairly recently in order for a person to have time off work with illness, it was necessary to have a doctor confirm that the patient was ill and therefore unable to attend work. This was an important social role in that it removed the responsibility from the worker and made legitimate this absence (Field 1976). This also increased the moral and authoritarian role of the doctor in society. This role has continued in the workplace, whereby a medical practitioner may be involved in the health aspects of employing and discharging employees. In the area of work surrounding medical fitness for work, i.e. medical examinations, returning to work following long-term absence, the occupational health physician will examine the person, and give a medical opinion to the employer who will decide whether the employment of the person will continue or not. Behaviour could be the dominant activity which is affecting the person's health; however, there may not be anything physical to measure.

This can be seen in mental illness where people demonstrate obsessive behaviour, or where people are experiencing occupational or personal stress and may be smoking and drinking to excess. Some people in jobs which are related to emergency services, such as fire services, may be experiencing post-traumatic stress. Whilst there may be physiological, mental and personality symptoms, not all need to be present (McCloy 1992). In addition to the trauma suffered by employees in stressful jobs is the organisational code which can put even more pressure onto employees:

> 'One of the biggest problems is that stress is still thought of as a weakness. Rescue personnel are often reluctant to admit to symptoms in case colleagues think that they are "softies".'
>
> (McCloy 1992, p. 163)

This phenomenon is also described by Duckworth (1991) in his paper on managing psychological trauma in the police service.

Control in organisational health could be seen as a way of protecting the individual from the harmful effects of the workplace. Not to have control measures could result in many more people suffering from occupational disease and injury. There have been examples in the USA where this control has infringed the civil liberties of workers. An example of which would be the situation where women who were working on a lead process were told that unless they had a sterilisation operation which would prevent them from becoming pregnant, they could no longer be permitted to do that job (Ellicott 1990). A more recent interesting development was the employee who successfully sued his employer for neglect. This was John Walker, a senior social worker for Northumberland County Council, responsible for four social work teams. Mr Walker had a nervous breakdown, but on his return to work he found that no concession had been made for him, and that his work load had increased. He asked for help, this was refused. Mr Walker suffered a second and more profound breakdown, which resulted in the Council dismissing him on the grounds of permanent ill-health (Howard 1995). Mr Walker won his case for negligence.

Physical health in the workplace

Exercise and fitness should, of course, be seen as aspects of prevention of sickness and injury, as well as promotion of wellbeing. It is also an opportunity for a type of work socialisation. Many organisations are actively encouraging a corporate approach to fitness. Evidence seems to be emerging that people who take regular exercise and are fit have less absenteeism from work when compared to other employees, and have a greater sense of satisfaction with their work (Shephard 1983; Ashton 1989). Employers in Japanese organisations manage the working day in such a way that there are exercise breaks at the beginning of the day and during the day. Everyone takes part in these exercises. This could be interpreted as paternalistic, but it does make good sense to ensure that people think about their bodies and its capabilities during the working day. An employer's major asset is the workforce; and all employers are morally and legally duty bound to care for employees whilst they are at work.

For many years some large organisations offered sports facilities; these tended to reflect the major sports interests of the time, i.e. football, rugby. Some organisations provided sports and social centres; these were usually an outdoor sports field and a social club for drinking and other social activities such as darts, card games, and dancing. With the changing times and current economic constraints, sports fields have tended to be sold off for their land value and arrangements made for more space conserving activities, i.e. gym work. Nationally, many organisations have taken on board the American pattern of providing exercise and health support systems in the workplace, some examples are Rank Xerox, IBM, Kellogg, Ford and Shell. All these companies provide corporate gymnasiums with professional instructors, essential for appropriate use of facilities (Bamford 1995).

Patterns of working in organisations

The 24-hour biological clock which regulates the body gives us our peak performance in the afternoon and our lowest performance between one and five in the morning (Harma 1992). Impaired health and shift work is discussed by many authors (Folkard 1987; Harrington 1978). There are few conclusive findings beyond gastrointestinal disorders (Harma 1992) and a general feeling of malaise likened to feelings of jet-lag.

However, Harma (1992), in a review of shift workers in Finland, found that shift workers:

> 'have twice the day worker's risk of stomach and duodenal ulcers. Moreover, the incidence of cardio-vascular disorders is increasing in shift workers.'
>
> (Harma 1992, p. 34)

Harma found that shift workers periodically suffered sleep disturbances, and for up to 25% this was a chronic situation.

British industry and the health care sector work a variety of shift patterns: regular days, 6 AM to 2 PM; afternoon shift, 2 PM to 10 PM; and nights, 10 PM to 6 AM. These shifts are often worked on a rotating basis, on a weekly rota, with weekends being free. Sometimes the shifts are worked for seven days or nights, and then two days off are taken; this is called a continental shift pattern having its origins in Europe.

Most employers require employees to work shifts in order to gain maximum output from machinery or because of the nature of the business requires 24-hour cover. Currently shift patterns in the NHS are causing concern. The human resources in an organisation are very costly. When those human resources are highly trained, more expense is incurred if they are not deployed and utilised effectively. The appropriate shift pattern to maximise those resources has been a debate in nursing for some years. The problem of shift working is emotive and of prime concern to the NHS, perhaps more so than other industries (Pownall 1990; Roscoe & Haig 1990). Any shift pattern which has the potential for disturbing normal sleep patterns has the potential for upsetting some individuals (Folkard 1987). Individuals who work shift rotation will have a disturbance to their normal sleeping patterns, which will have to be compensated for on their 'nights off' or rest days.

The effects of working at night can build up over many years, and it is probably a mix of factors rather than just the one variable of night work which causes ill effects (Folkard 1987). Any reading of the literature on shift working and health suggests that research is necessary (preferably longitudinal studies) to establish the reality for people doing this type of work (Brown 1988; Folkard 1987). There is a need also to study ex-shift workers. This group of workers was found by Harrington and Schilling (1981) to be more sickly than their colleagues who continued in shift work. The authors concluded that the underlying cause is unknown; however 20% of all people who start shift work have to give it up, and the most common reason is a medical one. Perhaps a medical reason is a more legitimate reason than not liking shifts or it being disruptive on family and social life. A person giving up shifts for medical reasons is more likely to be found alternative work than someone who just does not like, or is unable to work, shifts.

The greedy organisation

Just as working shift patterns can effect a person's wellbeing, working long hours can also have an effect. It seems that more organisations are expecting employees to work an increasingly long day, often not as overtime as it would have been in the past, but as part of a normal working pattern. As fewer people are employed to do the same or increased work then the people left in an organisation have little opportunity but to try to meet the demands of the work. Kanter (1989) in her discussion of workaholics and workforce exploitation, cites Coser (1974), and the concept of 'greedy organisations':

'ever-eager to consume more and more of the person, obliterating other choices, subordinating the rest of life to the demands of the company. By making the worker dependent on the rewards it holds out, the company can exact as much work as the person can bear, especially when the rewards include corporate status and power.'

(Kanter 1989, p. 269)

In some instances of course, attendance at work does not necessarily mean productivity. There is the phenomenon of being the first into the office and the last to leave, e.g. the notion that if one is always there then this must be a good thing. In Japan where hours of work and association with the organisation is legendary, a new illness is being described, *karoshi*, illness from overwork. McKee (1992) feels that this occurs because these people have little control over their working conditions, and gain very little achievement from that activity.

Sleep and employees' performance

Sleep is rarely mentioned in the health literature but there is increasing awareness of its importance, particularly in relation to performance, safety and decision making.

Hyyppa (1991) suggests that when considering strategies of sleep, sleep promotion and counselling need to be substantiated with scientific data rather than subjective and cultural approaches. There are suggestions that good sleepers seem to demonstrate qualities and attributes consistent with good or positive mental health.

Berrios and Shapiro (1993) feel that:

'About a third of people who go to see their general practitioners and about two-thirds of those who see psychiatrists complain that they are dissatisfied with the restorative quality of their sleep. Despite the size of these groups and the advances made by research workers, practical knowledge about the diagnosis and management of sleep-related complaints is limited'.

(Berrios & Shapiro 1993, p. 843)

Berrios and Shapiro feel that medical schools provide inadequate teaching about sleep disorders, and that many doctors hold the same beliefs about sleep disorders as their patients. These are often unsubstantiated and are thought to be secondary to some other condition or event. They feel that patients often blame recently developed fatigue, depression, irritability, tension, sleepiness, lack of concentration, drowsiness or muscular aches on the quality of their sleep. Sleep therefore is seen as important to individuals, but probably only as an indication of something else.

In a study by Jacquinet-Salord, *et al.* (1992) on sleeping tablet consumption, self-reported quality of sleep, and working conditions, the following conclusions were drawn:

'A high prevalence of self-reported sleep problems and related drug consumption was observed. Physical working conditions were not related to the quality of sleep in contrast to perceived job conditions. The results suggest that sleep quality might be a useful health indicator for the occupational physician.'

(Jacquinet-Salord 1992, p. 64)

This study was undertaken in 2769 small- to medium-sized firms in the Paris area. The study found no association between working conditions and sleep disturbances and drug consumption. The study was a large one, with a random sample of 7629 employees, 61% men and 39% women. People assessed their own quality of sleep; 16% of men and 26% of women said that they had sleep disturbances. One of the main reasons that people in this study took sleeping tablets was because of a 'bad atmosphere at work'.

In the study by Bamford (1993) a question was also asked about sleep, and in terms of sleep patterns: 298 people (55% of the sample) slept well; 92 (17%) experienced disturbed sleep patterns; 69 (13%) wakened early; 52 (10%) had difficulty getting to sleep and 26 (5%) had difficulty in waking up. This means that 45% of this sample were experiencing some abnormal sleep patterns. People could have responded to more than one category; the totals are shown in Table 3.3.

In this survey slightly more people (45%) were experiencing sleeping

Table 3.3 Sleep patterns.

Sleep pattern	Number of people
Slept well	298 (55%)
Disturbed sleep	92 (17%)
Waking early	69 (13%)
Difficulty getting to sleep	52 (10%)
Difficulty waking up	26 (5%)
Total	537 (100%)

difficulties than the sample surveyed by Jacquinet-Salord *et al.* (1992) in Paris. In that sample 42% of the people were experiencing self-reported sleep disturbance. However, the difference was not that great.

The comments on sleep given by people in Bamford (1993) to support their numerical score included:

'Stress, planning the next day's events, inability to switch off.'
'My wife died from cancer in March last year.'
'Mind too active, especially after shift work, body clock is always upset.'
'Stress of money.'
'Worry about work.'

These comments would be consistent with the comments made by individuals in this survey who were not experiencing good sleep and would be supported by Hyyppa's work on sleep (Hyyppa 1991), which is that people who feel their sleep is poor are likely to experience poor health.

Many people in Bamford's (1993) study used the word 'stress' to describe how they were feeling or to explain a behaviour such as disturbed sleep. They may just be people whose sleep is disturbed but for them that is the way it is. To call this behaviour stress is to give it a label which has some universality – people have a common understanding of it. It may not fit every clinician's understanding of the term, but it is useful to explain a disturbance between the individual and the environment which affects homeostasis, and for which there does not seem to be another explanation. However, this is restrictive in that it is applying the medical model to an event which may not be associated with disease, even though it may have an illness outcome.

Occupational and sickness absence

Sickness absence has been defined as absence from work which employees attribute to sickness or injury and which the employer accepts as such, (Baxter & Waldron 1989). Sickness absence in an organisation is really an indicator of people's absence from work and may or may not be associated with sickness. Absence from work is a multi-factoral issue. Women seem to have a higher rate of sickness absence than men and a greater proportion of short-term sickness absence than men, but they reported a lower percentage of health problems that limited their work than men. Younger and older workers also have a higher rate of sickness absences than other workers, with young people it is short-term absence, with older workers it is longer episodes of absence. 'A very high proportion of sickness absence spells are of less that 6 days, and the majority are in the 1–3 day category' (OPCS/HSE 1995, p. 227).

Research carried out at a Head Post Office in Wolverhampton (UK) indicated that:

> 'there was no statistically significant change in the frequency and severity of sickness absence, comparing two years before self-certification and three years after self-certification.'
>
> (Lim, 1985)

The employer is responsible for providing a financial safety net for employees who are off sick for ill health, whether the condition is occupationally related or not. The first three days are not covered by this net unless there is a contractual arrangement, but payment of some level for a period of up to 28 weeks is usually part of this agreement (Kloss 1989). The legislation covering this action here in the UK is the Social Security and Housing Benefits Act 1982 (DHSS 1982), and the Social Security Act 1985 (DHSS 1985).

Absenteeism has been a major problem to employers, as people could use the notion of sickness to absent themselves from work because that was seen socially as an acceptable thing to do. It was also a difficult area for a manager to challenge when the event was endorsed by a medical certificate issued by a GP. In the past that may have been the reason that some companies employed a doctor, to look over people who said they had been ill, and to challenge the medical decision of a peer. The changes in legislation affected this situation and made it legitimate for a manager to question absences from work whatever the cause (Taylor & Pocock 1981). When some large organisations began to monitor employees' sickness absence, there was a major reduction in sickness. An example of this is the considerable amount of work done by Peter Taylor who was the Medical Officer at the UK Post Office, which resulted in some instances of quite dramatic reductions in absence, and therefore increased productivity. Current work in this area of concern in the NHS and in other health care delivery systems is covered by such work as that carried out by Land (1993), Taunton *et al.* (1995) and Beil-Hildebrand (1996).

Managing for organisational health

It is important when managing for organisational health to remember the inter-related nature of activities in the workplace and in other aspects of a person's life. What happens at work is part of the totality of the individual, just as what takes place outside work is of equal importance. Leadership in the workplace is important as highlighted in the three dimensional model proposed by Bruhn and Chesney (1994), but they go on to say that 'it is a common myth that the leader determines an organisation's health and success'. They go on to cite Kelley's work (1992) in that 'a leader's effect on organisational success is only 10 to 20 percent: followership is the factor that makes for success' (Bruhn & Chesney 1994, p. 21–22). Interestingly they cite psychodynamics and the ability to repair broken relationships as having more impact on an organisation's health. It is not sufficient to play lip service to QWL, there needs to be a conscious effort to put those concepts into practice, as this has been shown to pay dividends (Townsend 1991; Churchill 1992; del Bueno 1993; and Peddicord-Whitley & Putzier 1994). It is also important to remember that all people at work, with very few exceptions, are employees, (including senior managers!) they may have an organisational role which gives them a greater influence in the hierarchy, but they remain employees. Health at work and organisational health is therefore everyone's responsibility.

References

Ashton, D. (1989) *The Corporate Health Care Revolution.* Routledge & Kegan Paul, London.

Bamford, M. (1993) *Aspects of Health amongst an Employed Population.* PhD Thesis, Aston University, Birmingham.

Bamford, M. (1995) Health promotion in the workplace. In: *Health Promotion: Theory and Practice* (ed. J. Kemm & A. Close), pp. 300–317. Macmillan, London.

Bamford, M. (1996) Public health in the workplace. *British Journal of Community Health Nursing,* **1** (1), 27–30.

Baxter, P.J. & Waldron H.A. (1989) The introduction and monitoring of occupational disease. In: *Occupational Health Practice* (ed. H.A. Waldron), 3rd edn. Butterworth, London.

Beil-Hildebrand, M. (1996) Nurse absence – the causes and the consequences. *Journal of Nursing Management* **4**, 11–17.

Berrios, G.E. & Shapiro, C.M. (1993) I don't get enough sleep, doctor. *British Medical Journal,* **306**, 843–6.

Blaxter, M. (1990) *Health and Life-style.* Tavistock/Routledge, London.

Board of Trade (1996) *Competitiveness – Creating the Enterprise Centre of Europe.* HMSO, London.

Brown, P. (1988) Punching the body clock. *Nursing Times,* **84**(44), 26–8.

Bruhn, J.G. & Chesney, A.P. (1994) Diagnosing the health of organizations. *Health Care Supervision,* **13**(2), 21–33.

del Bueno, D.J. (1993) Reflections on Retention, Recognition, and Rewards. *Journal of Nursing Administration,* **23**(10), 6–7, 41.

Churchill, M. (1992) Employees are also our customers. *American Nephrology Nurses Association Journal*, **19**(2), 152.

Collinson, D. (1994) Strategies of resistance: power, knowledge and subjectivity in the workplace. In: *Resistance and Power in Organizations* (eds J.M. Jermier, D. Knights & W.R. Nord), pp. 25–8.

Corbett, M.J. (1994) *Critical Cases in Organizational Behaviour*. Macmillan, London.

Coser, L. (1974) *Greedy Organizations. Patterns of Undivided Commitment*. Free Press, New York, NY.

DHSS (1982) *Social Security and Housing Benefits Act 1982*. HMSO, London.

DHSS (1985) *Social Security Act 1985*. HMSO, London.

DoH (1989) *Working for Patients*. Cm 555. HMSO, London.

Duckworth, D.H. (1991) Managing psychological trauma in the police service: from the Bradford fire to the Hillsborough crush disaster. *Journal of Social and Occupational Medicine*, **41**, 171–3.

Efraty, D. & Sirgy, M.J. (1990) The effects of quality of working life on employee behavioural responses. *Social Indicators Research*, **22**, 31–47.

Ellicott, S. (1990) Fertile women need not apply. *The Times*, 31 October, 18.

Ferlie, E., Fitzgerald, L. & Ashburner, L. (1994) The creation and evolution of the new health authorities: the challenge of purchasing. *Health Services Management Research*, **7**(2), 120–30.

Ferlie, E. & Pettigrew, A. (1996) Managing through networks: some issues and implications for the NHS. *British Journal of Management*. **7** (Special Issue), S81–S99.

Field, D. (1976) The social definition of illness. In: *An Introduction to Medical Sociology* (ed. D. Tuckett), pp. 334–6. Tavistock Publications Ltd, London.

Flanagan, H. & Spurgeon, P. (1996) *Public Sector Managerial Effectiveness: Theory and Practice in the National Health Service*. Open University Press, Buckingham.

Flannery, R.B. (1990) *Becoming Stress Resistant Through the Project SMART Program*. Crossroad Publishing, New York.

Folkard, S. (1987) Circadian rhythms and hours of work. In: *Psychology at Work* (ed. P. Warr), 3rd edn. Penguin Books Ltd, London.

Handy, C. (1989) *The Age of Unreason*. Arrow Books, London.

Harma, M. (1992) Hard day's night for shift workers. *Work Health Safety*. Institute of Occupational Health, Finland.

Harrington, J.M. (1978) *Shift Work and Health: A Critical Review of the Literature*. HMSO, London.

Harrington, J.M. & Schilling, R.S.F. (1981) Work and health. In: *Occupational Health Practice* (ed. R.S.F. Schilling), pp. 47–72. Butterworth, London.

Harpaz, I. (1989) Non-financial employment commitment: a cross-national comparison. *Journal of Occupational Psychology*, **62**, 147–50.

Health and Safety Commission (1991) *Annual Report 1990/91*. HMSO, London.

Heerwagen, J.H., Henbach, J.G., Montgomery, J. & Weimer, W.C. (1995) Environmental design, work and well being. *American Association of Occupational Health Nurses Journal*, **43**(9), 458–68.

Holland, J.W. (1994) *A Doctor's Dilemma – Stress and the Role of the Carer*. Free Association Books, London.

Howard, G. (1995) Stress and the law. *Occupational Health*, **47**(2), 58–60.

Hyyppa, M.T. (1991) Promoting good sleep. *Health Promotion International*, **6**(2), 103–10.

Jacobson, S.F. & McGrath, H.M. (1983) *Nurses Under Stress*. John Wiley & Sons, New York.

Jacquinet-Salford, M.C., Kang, T., Fouriaud, C., Nicoulet, I. & Bingham, A. (1992) Sleeping tablet consumption, self-reported quality of sleep, and working conditions. *Journal of Epidemiology and Community Health*, **47**, 64–8.

Kanter, R.M. (1989) *When Giants Learn to Dance*. Simon & Schuster, London.

Kelley, R. (1992) *The Power of Followership*. Doubleday, New York, NY.

Kerce, E.W. & Booth-Kewley, S. (1993) Quality of working life surveys in organizations. In: *Improving Organizational Surveys: New Directions, Methods and Applications* (eds P. Rosenfield, J.E. Edwards & M.D. Thomas), pp. 188–209. Sage, London.

Kloss, D. (1989) *Occupational Health Law*. Blackwell Science, Oxford.

Land, L.M. (1993) Selecting potential nurses: a review of the methods. *Nurse Education Today*, **13**, 30–39;.

Lim, L. (1985) *Comparison of Patterns of Sickness Absence Before and After Self Certification Amongst Postmen in a Head Post Office*. MSc thesis. Aston University, England.

Loscocco, K.A. & Roschelle, A.R. (1991) Influences on the quality of work and nonwork life: two decades in review. *Journal of Vocational Behaviour*, **39**, 182–225.

McCloy, E. (1992) Management of post-incident trauma: a fire service perspective. *Occupational Medicine*, **42**, 163–6.

McKee, V. (1992) Workaholics of the world unite. *The Times*, 8 May, 5.

Macmurray, J. (1935) *Reason and Emotion*. Faber & Faber, London.

Makin, P., Cooper, C. & Cox, C. (1996) *Organizations and the Psychological Contract – Managing People at Work*. British Psychological Society, Leicester.

Maslow, A.H. (1954) *Motivation and Personality*. Harper, New York.

Meusz, C. (1995) Occupational health: dealing with stress. *Nursing Standard*, **10**(2), 27–30.

Mirvis, P.H. & Lawler, E.E. III. (1984) Accounting for the quality of working life. *Journal of Occupational Behaviour*, **5**, 197–212.

Morgan, G. (1986) *Images of Organization*. Sage, London.

Newton, T., Handy, J. & Fineman, S. (1995) *'Managing' Stress: Emotion and Power at Work*. Sage, London.

NHS (1990) The NHS and Community Care Act. HMSO, London.

Oatley, K. (1992) *Best Laid Schemes: The Psychology of Emotions*. University of Cambridge Press, Cambridge.

OPCS/HSE (1995) *Occupational Health Decennial Supplement*. HMSO, London.

Orbach, S. (1994) *What's Really Going on Here? Making Sense of Our Emotional Lives*. Virago Press, London.

Peddicord-Whitley, M. & Putzier, D-J. (1994) Measuring nurses' satisfaction with the quality of their work and work environment. *Journal of Nursing Care Quality*, **8**(3), 43–51.

Pollock, K. (1988) On the nature of social stress: production of a modrn mythology. *Social Science & Medicine*, **26**, 381–92.

Poulton, E.C. (1978). Blue collar stressors. In: *Stress at Work* (eds C.L. Cooper & R. Payne). John Wiley & Sons, Chichester.

Pownall, M. (1990). Shifting ground. *Nursing Times*, **86**(44), 19.

Putnam, L.L. & Mumby, D.K. (1993). Organizations: emotion and the myth of rationality. In: *Emotion in Organizations* (ed. S. Fineman), pp. 36–57. Sage, London.

Ransome, P. (1996) *The Work Paradigm – A Theoretical Investigation of the Concepts of Work*. Avebury, Aldershot.

Roscoe, J. & Haig, N. (1990) Planning shift patterns. *Nursing Times*, **86**(38), 31–3.

Shephard, R.J. (1983) Employees' health and fitness: the state of the art. *Preventive Medicine*, **12**, 644–53.

Smith, J.C. (1993) *Understanding Stress and Coping*. Macmillan Publishing Company, New York.

Spurgeon, P. & Barwell, F. (1995) The quality of working life: occupational stress, job satisfaction and well-being at work. In: *Work and Health* (ed. M. Bamford), pp.; 101–30. Chapman & Hall, London.

Sutherland, V.J. & Cooper, C.L. (1990). *Understanding Stress – A Psychological Perspective for Health Professionals*. Chapman & Hall, London.

Swan, E. (1994) Managing emotions. In: *Women in Management: a Developing presence* (ed. M. Tanton), pp. 80–109. Routledge, London.

Taunton, R.L., Hope, K., Woods, C.Q. & Bott, M.J. (1995) Predictors of absenteeism among hospital staff nurses. *Nursing Economics*, **13**(4), 217–29.

Taylor, P.J. & Pocock, S.J. (1981) Sickness absence – its measurement and control. In: *Occupational Health Practice* (ed. R.S.F. Schilling), pp. 339–58. Butterworth, London.

Toffler, A. (1980) *The Third Wave*. Collins, London.

Townsend, M.B. (1991). Creating a better work environment: measuring effectiveness. *Journal of Nursing Administration*, **21**(1), 11–14.

Turnbull, J. (1995) Hitting back at the bullies. *Nursing Times*, **91**(3), 24–7.

Warr, P. (1982) A national study of non-financial employment commitment. *Journal of Occupational Psychology*, **55**, 297–312.

Willcox, R. (1994) Positive mental and physical health screening at work. In: *Creating Healthy Work Organizations* (eds C.L. Cooper & S. Williams), pp. 49–74. John Wiley & Sons, Chichester.

Williams, S. (1994) Creating healthy work organizations. In: *Creating Healthy Work Organizations* (eds C.L. Cooper & S. Williams), pp. 7–24. John Wiley & Sons, Chichester.

WHO (1985) *Targets for Health for All. Targets in support of the European Regional Strategy for health for all*. World Health Organization, Copenhagen.

Part II
KEY CONCEPTS IN QUALITY, FINANCE AND INFORMATION MANAGEMENT

4
Quality Management in Health Care and Health Care Education

Ann Close

This chapter examines the ways in which quality management has evolved over the last decade and discusses the influences that politics, education, the professions, consumers and quality gurus have had on its subsequent development and practice. It also considers the impact contracting for health care has had on service and education providers here in the UK. It provides information on how to plan and develop a systematic approach to quality management by following a strategic planning cycle. The suggested action plan provides the reader with information and strategies on how to identify and maintain good quality. The discussion on evaluation processes can also be used to monitor the effects of management interventions. Readers who require a broad-based introduction to quality concepts and activities (or alternatively, a succinct revision of the techniques involved) will find the final focused section of the reading particularly helpful.

It could be argued that quality management depends as much on people as it does on systems and techniques (Øvretveit 1992). As the same author also states, however, there is a danger that systems such as standard setting, audit, BS 5750 and so on, may be more easily adopted in a bureaucratic culture like the British National Health Service (NHS) than the cultural changes which can only be achieved through enabling people to think about the way they do their work.

Systematic approaches to improving quality can, and do, often act as catalysts for change – providing frameworks which enable individuals to review their practices and reshape them accordingly. In order to sustain such quality improvements, these approaches themselves are required to undergo a process of adaptation and change. One only has to review historical developments in quality management (for example, quality control and statistical process control, standardisation, quality circles, and more recently approaches to reviewing processes such as business process re-engineering (e.g. Hammer & Champy

1993), to see that all the different models and frameworks used work towards the common goal of continuously improving the product or service. In health care we have seen various initiatives come and go, with varying degrees of acclaim and practical utility. Quality management is, however, also dependent on managing the process of change, and is therefore by its nature required to be responsive and dynamic. New systems and frameworks may seem to provide the ultimate panacea for our perceived ills, although in reality, most approaches have limited shelf-life. For this reason, and in the interests of this book's own shelf-life, the approaches discussed are those that have sustained the test of time; they are what we would like to describe as 'classical' approaches to quality improvement. In our view students who have grappled with the conflicting tenets and constructions of 'quality' will welcome this pragmatic approach to the literature, and find material of real value here with which to tackle their quality-related problems.

The evolution of quality management

There are a number of factors that have influenced the evolution of quality management over the last decade: politics, education, the professions, consumers and experts.

Political influences

Since its inception in 1948 the National Health Service has been striving towards its primary objective to achieve the effective and efficient delivery of care. The creation of the NHS saw determined efforts to collect reliable, consistent and comparable data on activity and costs. According to Jowett and Rothwell (1988), however:

> 'no attempt was made to draw useful conclusions from any of this data and many argued that the very process of data collection had become an end in itself.'

A situation which some would say has not changed even today.

Over the years there have been a number of major reorganisations (DHSS 1972a, 1979a) established to improve efficiency and effectiveness, but these have had little real impact (DHSS 1979a).

Management enquiry
Following the election of the Conservative government in 1979 it became apparent that many public sector organisations were considered to be

inefficient and lacked the more effective private sector management techniques. As a result a team led by Sir Roy Griffiths, managing director and deputy chairman of Sainsbury's, conducted an enquiry into NHS management here in the UK. The subsequent report accused the NHS of failing to address issues of quality management and suggested there was little evaluation of performance and practice or measurement of health output, and little assessment of whether the service met the population's needs (DHSS 1983, p. 10, para. 2). Subsequently all health authorities were expected to make quality a priority. This proved to be a significant impetus for the current upsurge in quality activities in health care.

NHS reforms

More recently reforms to health care organisations introduced in 1990 intended to address the issue of quality by the introduction of competition. These reforms were derived from three white papers, *Promoting Better Health* (DoH 1987), *Working for Patients* (DoH 1989b) and *Caring for People* (DoH 1989a) which preceded the NHS and Community Care Act (1990). The aim of the reforms was to raise the standard of health and health care and improve the efficiency and effectiveness of the health service by:

- Creating internal markets and a new system of contractual funding.
- Making new arrangements for allocating resources, including GP fund-folding, and allocations made on a weighted capitation basis.
- Providing better management at all levels of the NHS, with an emphasis on devolved decision making.
- Involving clinicians more in managing the resources.
- Placing greater emphasis on information giving, health promotion and disease prevention, and patient choice.

The Patient's Charter

The government launched the Patient's Charter in 1991 to act as a catalyst to the development of quality (DoH 1991). For the first time national rights and standards were made explicit and this enabled users of the health service to understand what they could expect from the health service (see Table 4.1).

Since then there has been encouragement for health and social services to draw up local charters (DoH 1995). Recently there has been a revision and updating of the original Patient's Charter now called *The Patient's Charter and You* (DoH 1995). This includes specific standards for:

- GP services
- hospital services

- community services
- ambulance services
- dental, optical and pharmaceutical services
- maternity services.

Table 4.1   Patient's Charter rights and standards

Existing Charter rights (pre-1992)

- To receive health care on the basis of clinical need, regardless of ability to pay.
- To be registered with a GP.
- To receive emergency medical care at any time.
- To be referred to an acceptable consultant and have a second opinion.
- To be given a clear explanation of any treatment proposed.
- To have access to health records.
- To choose whether to take part in medical research and medical student training.

New rights from April 1992

- To be given detailed information on local health services, including quality standards and maximum waiting times.
- To be guaranteed admission for treatment within two years.
- To have complaints investigated and a prompt written reply from the chief executive.

Charter standards from April 1992

These relate to:
- Respect for privacy, dignity, and religious and cultural beliefs.
- Arrangements to ensure people with special needs can use the services.
- Information to relatives and friends.
- Waiting time for an ambulance service.
- Waiting time for initial assessment in accident and emergency departments.
- Waiting time in outpatients.
- Cancellation of operations.
- A named, qualified nurse, midwife or health visitor responsible for each patient.
- Discharge of patients from hospital.

There has also been the release of the Maternity Charter (DoH 1994a) and a Children's Charter is also planned. These charters aim to put the patient first and to make clear to members of the public and health service staff the standards that ought to be reached.

There is no doubt that the Patient's Charter has had a significant impact. Patients generally are more aware of their rights, particularly with regard to waiting times for first appointments and in outpatient clinics and accident and emergency departments. This is evident in the increase in number of complaints received. However, in some cases patients' expectations are seen to be unrealistic by health professionals who are trying to contend with increasing demands on their time and seemingly diminishing resources.

There has also been a significant improvement in waiting times for treatment. According to the Patient's Charter (DoH 1995) in March 1991 over 50 000 patients were waiting 2 years or more to go into hospital. Now in parts of the country waiting time is less than 9 months.

Waiting times for outpatient clinic appointments and waiting times at the clinics have also improved. Although this has been achieved partly by reorganising the way in which clinics are run, it has also necessitated greater numbers of patients being seen more quickly. This provides the government with its desired rhetoric but provides considerable dissatisfaction to patients and professionals who feel that the quality of the consultation is lacking, in particular the time to ask questions and discuss personal concerns.

The updated Patient's Charter has caused difficulties for other reasons. Some standards were introduced with immediate effect and this did not give providers of health care time to make preparations to begin to meet these standards which raised misconceptions and unrealistic expectations. This has been particularly so with the standards relating to single-sex wards and washing and toilet facilities.

There have been mixed-sex wards in hospitals for many years in an effort to be cost effective. Many hospitals, even some of the newer ones built during the last decade, have inadequate washing and toilet facilities which cannot be rectified overnight. All health professionals support the need for privacy and dignity, but can only work with the facilities and resources they have. Although it is important to acknowledge the demands of the public for specific facilities these have to be within the organisation's ability to provide them and therefore the purchaser's ability to fund them.

The Patient's Charter has also given a focus to performance management. Data are collected monthly and quarterly on many of the standards. Results are incorporated into performance league tables for comparisons to be made between providers and these are published to enable the public to find out how successful their local provider is compared to others. There is concern that this approach emphasises activity and quantity as a measure of quality, whereas patients and staff are frequently more concerned about the quality processes and outcomes involved in health care.

The Department of Health and the Audit Commission
The Department of Health frequently produces guidelines, reports and other documents which help to influence the quality of patient care. The Audit Commission became responsible for the external audit of the NHS in October 1990. As well as reviewing the financial accounts the Commission's auditors have a duty to examine the economy, efficiency and

effectiveness of health organisations' use of resources. Each year several topics are selected for these value-for-money studies in both health care and education. A selection of these are listed in Table 4.2.

Table 4.2   Department of Health, NHS Executive and Audit Commission, reports and guidelines

Department of Health (DoH)
  Measuring the Quality – Nursing Care Audit 1990
  The Evolution of Clinical Audit 1994
  The Patient's Charter 1991
  The Patient's Charter and You 1995
  A Vision for the Future – The Nursing, Midwifery and Health Visiting Contribution
    to Health and Health Care 1993

NHSME/NHSE
  Framework of Audit for Nursing Services 1991
  Professional Advice for Purchasers. A DHA Project Discussion Paper 1991
  Purchasing for Health – A Framework for Action 1993
  Quality and Contracting. Taking the Agenda Forward 1994
  Clinical Involvement in Contracting. A Handbook of Good Practice 1995

Audit Commission
  The Virtue of Patients – Making the Best Use of Ward Nursing Resources 1991
  Measuring Quality. The Patient's View of Day Surgery 1991
  All in a Day's Work. An Audit for Day Surgery in England and Wales 1992
  Making Time for Patients – A Handbook for Ward Sisters and Their Managers
    1992
  Lying in Wait. The Use of Medical Beds in Acute Hospitals 1992
  Children First. A Study of Hospital Services 1993
  Taking Care – Progress with Care in the Community 1993
  What Seems to be the Matter – Communication between Hospitals and Patients
    1993
  Setting the Records Straight. A Study of Hospital Medical Records 1995

World Health Organization (WHO)
The World Health Organization is a supporter of the need for quality assurance in health care and recommends the development of programmes to increase the knowledge and skills required (WHO 1985a). Target 31 in *Targets for Health for All,* encourages all member states to have by 1990:

'built effective mechanisms for ensuring quality of patient care within their health care systems.'

(WHO 1985b)

Although the UK is part way to achieving this it cannot be said that this target has been achieved yet.

Educational influences

In the nursing, physiotherapy and occupational therapy professions, statutory bodies are responsible for standards of education. In nursing the UKCC discharges this function through four national bodies which are required to make provision for nurse education and training, approve institutions and courses, arrange examinations and promote improved training. In physiotherapy it is the Chartered Society of Physiotherapists and in occupational therapy, the College of Occupational Therapy that undertake this role. In the medical professions, the Royal Colleges are responsible for standards of post-registration education, in conjunction with postgraduate deans and clinical tutors, who are also responsible for managing related budgets.

In nursing, for decades there have been frequent expressions of concern over declining standards, with a variety of solutions suggested (RCN 1943; Ministry of Health 1947; DHSS 1972b). More recently the Merrison report (DHSS 1979b) related the problems to 'untrained staff left in charge of wards, unsupervised learners and increased workload', all of which suggest a neglect of students' preparation.

Research studies have uncovered aspects of the clinical environment which appeared to be inconsistent with learning (Fretwell 1982; Alexander 1983; Gott 1983; Reid 1985). These studies demonstrated that little teaching was done, with tutors teaching 'ideal' rather than 'real' care.

Many of these reports gave recommendations and guidance on how to improve the quality of education but were often ignored or deemed to be unsuitable in the prevailing political climate. Some of these issues started to be addressed with the introduction of Project 2000 training which attempts to produce flexible, critically aware practitioners who can respond to unpredictable health care demands of the 1990s and beyond.

Further changes are occurring as nurse and midwifery education is integrated into higher education institutions to further improve the academic quality of programmes delivered. This will help to bring it in line with many of the other health care professionals, such as physiotherapists and occupational therapists, who currently have pre-qualification education in universities with the statutory bodies ensuring there are consistent standards across the country. Within higher education there are many mechanisms which have been used to ensure quality and maintenance of academic standards, including course accreditation regulations, peer review, external examiners and by using a number of performance indicators such as financial indicators, examination successes and the number of research papers produced.

Much of the non-medical education occurring in higher education is commissioned by health service organisations and this enables quality specifications and monitoring to be incorporated into the contracting process which will be discussed later.

Professional influences

Statutory bodies

The majority of health professional groups have regulatory bodies responsible for maintaining professional standards and professional conduct. For example, in nursing, midwifery and health visiting the United Kingdom Central Council (UKCC) maintains a register of qualified practitioners. It lays down a code for the conduct of professionals which recognises the relationship between accountability and standards of practice (UKCC 1992). It also protects patients from ineffective and unscrupulous practitioners. The General Medical Council has a similar function in relation to medical practitioners as does the Chartered Society of Physiotherapists and the College of Occupational Therapy for physiotherapists and occupational therapists respectively.

Professional bodies such as the Royal Colleges of Nursing and Midwifery, all the medically related colleges and the organisations for occupational therapists and physiotherapists undertake work aimed at improving the quality of patient care. An example is the work undertaken by the Royal College of Nursing on quality assurance and standard setting over the last decade in the Standards of Care project.

Consumer influences

Consumers have had an increasing influence on health care provision over the last twenty years.

Community Health Councils

Community Health Councils (CHC) were set up as a result of the 1973 NHS Reorganisation Act. Their main functions have been to review the operation of the health service, make recommendations for improvement and to provide a way of helping the public make their views known to health authorities.

Under the regulations members have made visits to local hospitals and community units and have made recommendations based on the findings made during such visits. They frequently undertake projects focused on particular aspects of the health service from a consumer's standpoint. This may be in conjunction with Trusts or other provider units, for example studies on access to hospital premises from a disabled person's perspective.

CHCs have few formal powers and try to influence through advice and persuasion, a situation which has been made more difficult by the NHS reforms and the establishment of Trusts.

The media

The media have provided the public with more information about the health service. A day rarely goes by without some health care issue making the news headlines. Women's magazines publish articles about health, and radio and television programmes frequently seek the views of audiences on health service provision. This raises people's awareness and expectations of the type and quality of health services and provides them with a means of lobbying for an increase, or improvement in those services.

Voluntary organisations

Voluntary organisations, such as the National Association for the Welfare of Children in Hospital, the National Childbirth Trust and many others, are able to exert pressure on health service organisations in order to make changes.

Patients' representatives

Consumer relations officers or patients' representatives have been appointed in a number of hospitals. In July 1992 the NHS Management Executive (NHSME) funded a project designed to look at the role of the patients' representative. The aim of having a patients' representative is to listen to patients' views about the kind of care they want and to develop services which are less bureaucratic and more friendly to patients.

Patients' representatives are beneficial in helping to sort out patients' concerns, providing an independent view, acting as an identified person who knows the hospital and can get things done by solving problems and negotiating across departments and directorates (McIver 1993).

Expert influences

There are many individuals who have had a significant impact on developing and introducing approaches to quality. Many of these began in industry and have since had some impact in the public sector and the health service. The work of three such experts is considered briefly.

W. Edwards Deming

Deming focused on statistical quality control methods initially and introduced a PDCA cycle – *P*lan, *D*o, *C*heck and *A*ction – to improve quality. This emphasises the importance of action planning, setting goals and ways of meeting them, and engaging in education and training before implementing the work, checking the effects of implementation, and finally, taking appropriate action.

Deming developed a 14 point action plan for change applicable to any industry for quality improvement to be successful (Walton 1986). These points advocate involving staff in making decisions, team-working, improving communication across departments, effective leadership and supervision, education, improved relationships between management and staff, and focusing on quality and effective processes rather than finance and activity.

In later years he developed the concept of quality and management activity and recognised the contribution that employees can make through their understanding of the processes and how they can be improved.

Philip Crosby

A particularly significant contributor to the debate on quality is Philip Crosby and although his work has been developed in industry many of the principles he proposes are relevant, and have had some influence, in health care and education settings.

Crosby (1979) maintains that:

'Quality is an achievable, measurable, profitable, entity that can be installed once you have commitment and understanding and are prepared for hard work.'

He advocates dispelling the myths that 'quality means goodness', 'error is inevitable' and 'people lack concern for their work'. Instead, he believes, quality is conformance to requirements. It is cheaper to do things right first time and employees have the best ideas about why things were done wrong the first time.

Crosby supports the view that there should be a corporate-wide emphasis on quality which requires:

- *Management participation* – all managers should feel that participation in the quality programme is routine and expected.
- *Professional quality management* – there are individuals who are freed organisationally to undertake quality measurements.
- *Original programmes for quality improvement* – programmes that are going to fire the enthusiasm of those who are involved.
- *Recognition* – for people who offer outstanding support to quality programmes.

Dr Joseph M. Juran

Juran's focus is on quality management from the top of the organisation. He identified eight success factors which characterise organisations that have improved quality (Juran 1988). In these organisations top managers had:

- Personally led the quality process.
- Adopted quality improvement plans with roles and responsibilities clearly identified.
- Involved all those affected.
- Trained management staff in quality planning, control and improvement.
- Trained the workforce to participate in quality improvement.
- Included quality improvement in strategic planning.
- Applied quality improvement to business planning and operational processes.
- Used modern quality methodology instead of empiricism in quality planning.

Juran (1989) organised quality management into three parts which he called a *quality trilogy*:

- *Quality planning*. This involves determining who the customers are and their needs and developing processes which result in products which respond to customer needs.
- *Quality control*. This requires evaluating product performance and comparing this to product goals and then acting on the differences.
- *Quality improvement*. This requires identifying improvement projects and establishing the projects teams with resources, training and motivation to diagnose the cause of problems, identify solutions and establish mechanisms to monitor and maintain progress.

The overriding message from these experts is that the management function is crucial in determining the quality of services and products. Health service staff are often suspicious and mistrust ideas that have come from industry as they believe that service providers which have people as their focus have different requirements from industries which manufacture products. This is undoubtedly true, but the principles used should be carefully considered because many can be adapted and adopted in diverse settings.

Purchasing quality health care and education

Contracting in health care

As a result of the NHS reforms (NHS 1990) all purchasers and provider units have been required to have contracts or service agreements since April 1991. Although, according to NHSME guidance (NHSME 1990d) service specifications should comprise descriptions of planned services and quality standards to be required by residents from current providers, there was some apprehension that price would be the dominating factor in the contracting process.

The emphasis initially was on maintaining planned levels of service, but the need:

'to begin to address quality standards e.g. in the priority areas of waiting lists and waiting times and maternity and neonatal services,'
(NHSME 1990d, p. 13)

was acknowledged. However, these examples in themselves have raised concerns that the focus of quality is on the quantity, activity and throughput elements *rather than* process and outcome aspects.

Contracts were expected to contain explicit standards against which the quality of services or care could be measured. Specifications may describe quality at a global level or be more detailed relating to individual elements of the service.

At present the way the majority of purchasers contract for health services is to agree on how many contacts staff will have with patients or how many finished consultant episodes (FCEs) there are. Quality clauses are usually added to the contract but have a varying effect on improving the quality of care.

Health care education

Similar approaches have also been taken in education. *Working Paper 10 – Education and Training* and subsequent guidance documents outlined the changes in the organisation and funding of non-medical education training which has resulted in the introduction of commissioning into health care education (NHSME 1990a; 1990b; 1990c; 1990e).

Initially, regional health authorities (RHAs) were responsible for allocating funds for non-medical education and training and in planning and assessing demand for, and in ensuring the supply of, training. Acting on behalf of Trusts and directly managed units (DMUs), they commissioned pre-qualifying education for many non-medical health professional groups and placed contracts with colleges of nursing and midwifery and other education establishments that provide health care education.

With the recent changes to the structure of NHS management and the abolition of RHAs as a result of the functions and manpower review, arrangements for commissioning pre-qualification education and training are changing. In future workforce planning and the determination of intake levels to training programmes will be the employer's responsibility. In practice this will be undertaken by consortia of NHS and non-NHS health care providers, GPs and purchasers. In addition consortia will take responsibility for budgets, commissioning and therefore contracting. An overview of this process will be made by Regional Education and Development Groups (NHSE 1995).

There have been many different arrangements for post-qualifying education and training. Working Paper 10 intended that post-qualification education should be, in general, funded and commissioned by employers except where it is:

'necessary to provide highly specialised skills and where the incidence of training costs is uneven.'

(NHSME 1990c)

However, some regions have played a commissioning role as in pre-qualification, in others each individual Trust or unit has commissioned its own post-qualification education and training.

In comparison to service contracts, a similar emphasis was placed on ensuring stability but this time, in the funding of existing training provision (NHSME 1990c). As contracting has developed there has been a focus on the quantitative elements, such as numbers of qualified professionals produced. The quality of courses has generally been left to the relevant statutory bodies, the Trusts and units concerned or the colleges themselves to address.

More recently though, there has been an increase in the specification of standards of quality.

Key issues in contracting

In the years since the introduction of contracts in health care and health care education there is no doubt that the contracting process has become more sophisticated. Nevertheless there are still some key issues which need to be addressed if quality is to be a driving force in the contracting process. Many of these issues have been identified in the National Health Service Executive (NHSE) Purchasing Unit document *Quality and Contracting. Taking the Agenda Forward* (NHSE 1994).

Quality of commissioning
The focus of quality in contracting to date has been almost exclusively
on the quality of services by provider units. However, in 1993 Dr
Mawhinney, as Minister of Health, identified key elements required for
successful purchasing. These include:

- *A strategic approach* – purchasers need to take a five-year forward
  look and give providers some ideas of purchasing intentions to enable
  them to plan effectively.
- *Effective contracts* – commissioners must ensure that services which
  are contracted on behalf of the population are of high quality and
  incorporate value for money.
- *Knowledge of the population's needs* – this is necessary for deciding
  on type and range of service to contract and the resources allocated
  to each.
- *Responsiveness to local people* – commissioners need to seek and act
  on views of public representatives.
- *Mature relationships with providers* – working with providers will
  help commissioners to develop detailed knowledge of what the service can actually offer.
- *Local alliances* – commissioners need to work with GPs, local
  authorities, voluntary bodies and others to create healthy environments and collaborative approaches to ensure health gain.
- *Organisation capacity* or organisational fitness.

Both Benton (1994) and Øvretveit (1994) recognise that commissioners share many of these responsibilities with providers for the
quality of providers' services and the NHSE (1994) offers guidance on
how to achieve a more collaborative approach.

Large numbers of quality standards
Provider units frequently have contracts with a large number of purchasers or commissioning teams including an increasing number of GP
fund-holders. It is not uncommon for each to produce its own set of
global and specific quality standards, which it requires the provider unit
to achieve. In some cases the quality specification from some purchasers
has a large number of standards, for example, in one case more than 260.
If this is multiplied by, for example, five main purchasers or more, then
provider units can be expected to have to address more than 1000 different standards. The benefits to patient care are questionable in such
situations.

The NHSE report (1994) suggests that one way forward might be for
neighbouring purchasing organisations to produce a small set of agreed

core quality standards which are meaningful to providers and which can be monitored regularly.

Monitoring arrangements and emphasis on outcomes
Some commissioners do not have effective monitoring mechanisms in place and this is often the case when there are large numbers of standards. In some cases some of the standards are virtually impossible to measure anyway.

To assist this situation the NHSE (1994) suggests having a core set of standards, using existing mechanisms, e.g. accreditation: focusing on clinical outcomes as well as processes, and for commissioners to have a clear purpose and added value in asking providers for more information. They also recommend that GPs work closely with health authorities on monitoring.

Clinical involvement in contracts
There are strong arguments for the involvement of clinical staff in the contracting process as they are the staff delivering care to patients. The NHSE (1994) report recognises the most significant stage for this involvement to be in the initial stages of shaping the contract, the delivery and review of the contract. The NHSE also recommends that the focus needs to move away from financial aspects and concentrate on improving effectiveness and quality of services to enhance the involvement of clinicians (NHSE 1995).

The need for a planned strategic approach

There is evidence to suggest that attempts to introduce quality assurance activities have often been haphazard and uncoordinated events. Over the last decade health care professionals have become increasingly aware of the need to provide good quality, cost-effective health care.

There are several reasons why this might have occurred. It may be due to traditional approaches being taken by health care staff which did not focus on the delivery of cost-effective services or the lack of preparation to participate in quality monitoring activities. Alternatively, in some cases, professional groups have been working in isolation, either omitting to involve colleagues or failing to gain their co-operation and support.

Another important reason, is that although quality may feature in the organisation's business plan it is often seen as an afterthought rather than an essential component. The message this gives to staff is that quality services are not as important as activity targets or finances and that they are an additional extra.

Other factors include lack of financial and human resources and a lack of commitment from managers. It is essential that there is management leadership to motivate and support staff in developing and implementing quality assurance activities and quality initiatives.

Quality is not a technique or task to do in addition to everything else. Instead it is a philosophy or way of doing something which is embodied into every aspect of the organisation's working life. If this is not the case then quality will be quickly seen as a fad, flavour of the month or just another bandwagon.

Creating quality requires an organisation to continually strive for excellence. It is important to focus on at least seven variables in the organisation: strategy, structure, people management style, systems and procedures guiding concepts and shared values, and the skills contained within the organisation. Peters and Waterman (1982) describe these variables as the McKinsey 7-S Framework.

These variables are interdependent and should not be considered in isolation, but in the past in the health service we have tended to pay more attention to the 'hard Ss' – strategy, structure and systems, with less consideration being given to the 'soft Ss' of style, staff, skills and shared values.

- **Strategy**
  In order to ensure effective management of quality, strategic planning is essential. The strategic plan provides a coherent set of actions aimed at giving the organisation a clear focus and direction. Strategic planning is a management tool which will ensure the long-term continuation and growth of quality initiatives and activities in an organisation such as a hospital, college of health studies or GP practice.

  In the past efforts to put things right have tended to be reactive, knee-jerk responses to problems, investigations and reports. Strategic planning is proactive and takes a long-term perspective as well as considering short-term issues. Strategies that succeed in the NHS are dynamic; they evolve, taking account of rapid changes in the health care environment, in shifting consumer expectations and demands set by purchasers.

- **Structure**
  This is the organisational chart showing how tasks are divided up and integrated, where individual and group responsibilities rest and who reports to whom.

- **Systems**
  These are the processes and procedures through which things get done on a day-to-day basis.

- **Staff**
  The people within the organisation, including individuals and groups, and how they are involved and contribute.

- **Skills**
  These are the capabilities possessed by the organisation as a whole.

- **Style**
  This is the way in which management presents itself to other employees, with respect to their use of time, what they give their attention to and their specific actions. It is also how the whole work force presents itself to the outside world.

- **Shared values**
  This is the fundamental philosophy that underpins the organisation.

Strategic plan

The strategic plan is a cyclical process (Fig. 4.1) which consists of four main phases which respond to the following questions:

Phase		*Question*
(1)	Diagnosis of current situation	Where are we now?
(2)	The vision, goals and targets	Where do we want to be?
(3)	The action plan	How will we get there?
(4)	Evaluation	
	Formative	How will we know we are getting there?
	Summative	How will we know when we get there?

This approach can be used in hospital, community and education settings, to plan activities for the organisation as a whole or wards, departments and teams.

Diagnosis of the current situation
It is essential to determine the starting point for quality and to consider the factors which influence the quality of work done by the organisation. It helps to identify clearly existing practices that are worthwhile and areas which need to be developed.

Information can be collected from a variety of sources:

- staff from various groups working at all levels of the organisation
- the organisation's business plan
- contracts

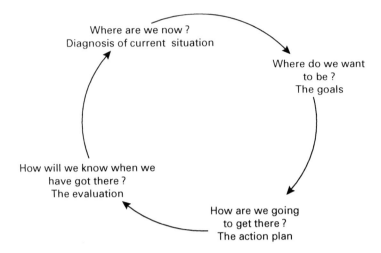

Fig. 4.1 The strategic cycle.

- internal and external reports, and other documents
- formal and informal meetings with colleagues
- experts or consultants to the organisation
- local and national policies and guidelines

The following areas should be explored to establish a baseline from which to work:

- **The organisation's business plan**
  This will identify the mission statement and philosophy which clarify the purpose and direction of the organisation, provide more detailed information about the organisation's values and beliefs and make explicit what qualities members of the organisation wish to pursue, monitor and evaluate. It will also provide details of the current service provision and future plans and therefore, sets the scene and directs the process for the delivery of quality services or education.

- **Characteristics of customers**
  It is important to determine who are the customers of the organisation as a whole, and of different departments; what services or products do you provide them with: what are their requirements and what do they think of the services? These will differ enormously, for example the needs of children compared to elderly people; pre-registration Project 2000 students compared to post-registration degree students.

- **Characteristics of the staff population**
  This should include a profile of the numbers, types and skills of staff

and what they understand about the functions and values of the organisation and quality assurance. Their views should be sought on a number of things such as:

- ○ the involvement of the unit in quality activities
- ○ the quality of the services they provide
- ○ current methods of quality assurance
- ○ the organisation and co-ordination of quality activities
- ○ the level of their contribution
- ○ their current knowledge and skills, what education and training they have had and where they need assistance in the future
- ○ the activities they want to see introduced in the future.

- **Current quality activities**
  A review of current activities will help to identify what is being done by which groups of staff. Those activities which are beneficial to service provision can be retained and developed in other areas and those which are not as effective can be changed or discontinued.

- **Resources and support**
  The availability of finances, equipment and human resources to use on quality development and monitoring and related activities such as staff education and training should also be established.

- **Culture, ethos and management style**
  An assessment of the management style should be made. An organisation which encourages and empowers staff to be more responsible and work in partnership requires a different approach to quality than one which is authoritarian and controlling.

- **SWOT**
  This first phase of the planning cycle can be completed with a SWOT analysis
  - ○ *strengths* of the organisation compared with competitors
  - ○ *weaknesses* of the organisation compared with competitors
  - ○ *opportunities* for the organisation in its environment
  - ○ *threats* to the organisation in its environment.
  Comparing the organisation with the performance in other organisations is increasingly important in the NHS market and this exercise will help to shape and develop quality services.

Additional factors influencing the quality strategy
There are also a number of external factors which may influence the development of a quality strategy. These will vary depending on the type of organisation or whether the quality strategy is being done for a specific part of the organisation. There will be national, regional and local

influences from government, professional bodies, purchasers, health and social service departments and education institutions, see Table 4.3 for examples.

Table 4.3 External influences in developing a quality strategy.

In an Acute Trust
The Patient's Charters
Quality specifications in purchaser contracts
Health of the Nation targets
The NHS reforms
The community care reforms
The new deal – junior doctors' hours
Priorities and planning guidance
Audit Commission reports

In an educational establishment
Integration of colleges into higher education institutions
Working Paper 10 and commissioning of education
Quality specifications in purchaser contracts
The NHS reforms
The community care reforms
Professional regulation
Trusts and other units, plans and strategies
Audit Commission reports

The vision and goals

People tend not to work well when they are unclear of the organisation's direction and their role within it. This phase of the planning cycle establishes a clear vision of where the organisation wants to be and identifies goals for quality. The goals should be linked to the organisation's business plan and should help members of staff understand what is expected of them. The goals also provide a yardstick by which the organisation can measure its success in achieving the strategy.

The goals should be:

- relevant to the work of the organisation
- measurable
- precise and understandable
- achievable
- consistent with the overall objectives of the organisation.

Spending time on goal setting at this stage, to achieve the above, will greatly assist evaluation (see Table 4.4).

Table 4.4   Goals for quality in an NHS Trust. Information from the Dudley Group of Hospitals (1995).

Target 1	*Quality culture, quality management* To develop a quality culture across the Trust and integrate quality into management processes.
Target 2	*Directorate quality improvement plans* Each directorate will develop, implement and evaluate an annual quality improvement plan and provide a report to the quality steering group.
Target 3	*Professional and clinical audit* To develop, implement and evaluate a programme of professional and clinical audit.
Target 4	*National and local Charter standards and purchaser's quality specifications* To meet the Patient's Charter targets and contract quality specifications set by the purchasers and the Trust.
Target 5	*Communication* To develop effective communication and information exchange about the quality of services with consumers.
Target 6	*Trust-wide quality initiatives* To introduce two Trust-wide quality initiatives aimed at improving patients and/or staff quality of life. (1) Health promoting hospitals. (2) Pressure sore prevention and management.
Target 7	*Training and developing for quality* To provide training and development opportunities and support to enable staff to undertake quality monitoring and improvement activities.

Developing and implementing the action plan

This phase describes the actions required to achieve the goals. It involves identifying the key tasks and actions that need to occur, who will do them, in what sequence and by what date.

Activities will vary depending on the current situation in the organisation and the vision it has of the future. Nevertheless there are always a number of challenges to face when developing and implementing the action plan and it is wise to consider alternative courses of action.

It is important to consider:

- How good quality will be identified.
- How it will be measured and monitored and whether there are any preformulated tools that can be used.

- How activities will be co-ordinated; are there any frameworks that will help this?
- How to achieve successful implementation and
  - get support from key people
  - motivate staff and get their commitment
  - make sure we get the work done.

There are many ways of approaching this and the ones used will vary depending on the needs of the organisation. It is likely that a combination of approaches may be considered.

Identifying good quality

Quality may be identified by means of national or local criteria which require checks to be in place to ensure that the specific criteria are maintained. These checks or *quality controls* may be carried out by external bodies or internally by staff in the organisation. In hospitals there are many examples, such as checking procedures for controlled drugs; checking qualifications of staff; daily calibration tests of laboratory equipment and fire safety checks. Similarly examples in education are validation of marking by external examiners and by using specific recruitment and selection criteria. The focus is on concurrent performance monitoring and correction.

An alternative approach is *quality assessment*. It is necessary to determine beforehand what you are going to look at, why and how you are going to do it. A predetermined standard or description of what is good is also required for comparison with the actual performance. Any discrepancies or deficiencies highlighted during the assessment are considered and ways of improving them are explored to result in *quality improvement*.

An example in education would be to survey a group of students to assess their views on a course or specific module and then to make changes as appropriate. Similarly an assessment of the quality of nursing documentation could be undertaken in a health care setting. Guidelines of good practice and additional training can be introduced to improve the quality of the documentation.

The repetition of quality assessment followed by quality improvement described above will ensure progress towards *quality assurance*.

A way of managing which sees quality as being fundamental to all the organisation's activities along with cost and quantity, is essential to support these activities. *Quality management* emphasises the need for continuous learning to maintain continuous improvement of services and requires good leadership, staff training and improvement of work and management processes. Crucial to the approach is recognition of staff members' contribution.

Maxwell's dimensions (1984)

Maxwell suggests there are six dimensions to quality which need to be recognised separately and which require different measures and assessment skills:

- access to service
- relevance to need
- effectiveness
- equity
- social acceptability
- efficiency and economy.

This approach has sometimes been used by purchasers in the quality specifications in contracts (see Table 4.5 for examples).

Table 4.5 Purchaser quality specifications using Maxwell's dimensions.

Access	Patients have reasonable access to services in terms of geographical convenience, waiting time for treatment, physical design of buildings, availability of transport.
Relevance to need	The services provided are appropriate to the needs of the local population.
Effectiveness	The services actually achieve the intended benefits and outcomes.
Equity	Services are even-handed between different patients and social groups.
Social acceptability	The service is provided in ways (including customer relations, style of service, flexibility, and impact on the community at large) which are acceptable to the population served.
Efficiency and economy	The service is provided in such as way as to give value for money.

Donabedian (1966)

Donabedian's approach to describing an organisation is based on the system's theory of input, throughput and output. When applied to the health care or education setting:

- *input* or *structure*   describes the resources required to deliver health care or education
- *throughput* or *processes*   describes the activities staff undertake
- *output* or *outcome*   describes the results or effects of health care interventions or changes in behaviour as a result of learning.

This approach has been used frequently in health care and health care education linked with Lang and Clinton's (1984) framework for change discussed later.

Quality tools

There are many different tools that can be used in health care and health care education and the following is a small selection. Similarities can be seen between some and some are used in conjunction with others.

Performance indicators
These are 'tools developed to measure and indicate the efficiency and effectiveness of an organisation' (RCN 1987). They consist of numerical values which assess aspects of a system. They were first introduced into the health service in the early 1980s and into health care education in 1983 (Balough & Beattie 1988; ENB 1986).

Performance indicators are used to assist managers to review systems and examine results and they highlight areas where questions need to be asked and investigations made. They can also be used to compare organisations. There are concerns that the indicators fail to do justice to the complexities of health care and education because they emphasise products at the expense of processes. In addition there are many aspects of an organisation's performance that cannot be reduced to such statistics (Yorke 1991).

Examples of performance indicators in health care are pressure sore prevalence indicators and infection rates; and in education, destination of graduates and wastage and completion rates.

Benchmarking
This is a process of seeking, finding, implementing and sustaining best practice. It can be done internally by comparing similar processes in different parts of the organisation, for example discharge of patients, or it can be used externally to compare the performance of different organisations in specific measurable terms, such as provision of domestic services.

Benchmarking concentrates on understanding processes and rectifying failure points in a system. It uses performance indicators and comparative databases to identify the performance gap and best practice.

Quality circles
Quality circles consist of groups of volunteer workers who are trained to identify, analyse and solve problems. The solution to the problem is then

implemented and monitored to establish if the problem has been solved (Osborne 1987; Sale 1990). The circle involves:

- problem identification
- selection of the problem for study
- analysis by circle and experts
- solutions
- implementation of chosen solutions
- presentation to management.

The circle requires:

- a co-ordinator to ensure the activity continues
- a facilitator to make sure the circle gets going and maintains its momentum
- a leader who will require special training in group dynamics, leadership, problem solving and quality circle philosophy
- a recorder to take notes of meetings.

Quality circles are useful because they involve staff in decision making and develop teamworking and interaction with others in the organisation. However, it requires training and as with most systems used it is time consuming to undertake and therefore costly.

Audit

This is a process which involves systematically looking at the work-related procedures and activities, and examining the use of associated resources and the effects this has on outcomes and quality for the user.

In health care, *clinical audit* is involved in

'systematically looking at procedures used for diagnosis, care and treatment, examining how associated resources are used and investigating the effect care has on the outcome and quality of life for the patient.'

(DoH 1994b)

Clinical audit should use a multidisciplinary approach and focus on patients and on improving clinical effectiveness and patient outcomes.

A similar process can be used in education to examine all the activities related to education, the related resources and the outcomes in terms of students' learning and development.

The audit cycle described above is very similar to the Dynamic Standards Setting System developed by the Royal College of Nursing (RCN 1990).

Models and frameworks

Having a framework or model will help to co-ordinate and provide structure to the varied activities being used.

Framework of Audit for Nursing Services (NHSME 1991)
This framework consists of three key components:

- *The audit square* which shows the main areas of nursing service in which audit can be carried out and the four component stages of audit: objective/standard setting; implementation; measurement and recording, and monitoring and action planning.
- The *audit classification* which allows adaptable issues to be grouped in a structured and logical way.
- The *audit form* which has the audit protocol for each issue. The protocol defines the focus, approach and method used for auditing each issue or topic.

This framework can be adapted for education settings (Close & MacNeil 1993) and can be used in multidisciplinary settings in hospitals and community services as well as for nursing services (see Figs 4.2a and 4.2b).

Wilson's adult learning model (1987)
Wilson's adult learning model was developed to introduce quality assurance into hospitals in Canada (Wilson 1987). It involves six steps:

(1) The documentation of existing quality management and quality activities in the organisation.
(2) The reporting and communicating of these activities to improve recognition of quality performances.
(3) The development of a quality assurance plan to incorporate existing and future activities.
(4) The developing and implementation of explicit standards and criteria.
(5) The development of criteria-based audits for all functions.
(6) The endorsement of all activities by a quality steering group.

This framework would also be appropriate in education because it recognises and uses mechanisms for assuring quality such as course validation and evaluation. In addition a wide range of new activities, such as standard setting and consumer surveys, can be introduced in a series of stages to build up to complete an overall plan which will then be related to the organisation's business plan.

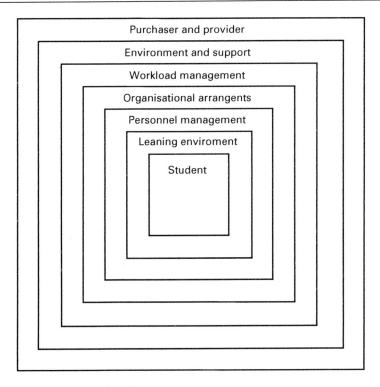

Fig. 4.2a   Audit square in education.

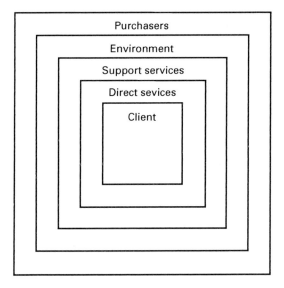

Fig. 4.2b   Audit square in a provider Trust.

Lang and Clinton (1984) – a framework for change
This model represents a continuous circular process for nursing quality
assurance and has 11 steps:

(1)　Identify and agree values.
(2)　Review literature and known quality assurance programmes.
(3)　Analyse available programmes.
(4)　Determine the most appropriate quality assurance programme.
(5)　Establish structure, process and outcome standards and criteria.
(6)　Ratify standards and criteria.
(7)　Evaluate current levels of nursing practice against ratified standards.
(8)　Identify and analyse factors contributing to results.
(9)　Select appropriate action to maintain and improve quality.
(10)　Implement selected action.
(11)　Evaluate quality assurance programme.

This model has been developed by the Royal College of Nursing (RCN)
as the dynamic standard setting system and incorporates Donabedian's
approach to the examination of an organisation and Lang's model of
quality assurance (RCN 1990). Although it was developed initially for
nursing, it has been widely used by many health professionals in many
settings.

How to achieve successful implementation of a quality strategy

Successful implementation requires managers to reduce resistance, thus
getting support from key people and motivating everyone concerned.

Reducing resistance
People resist new ideas and changes for a whole variety of reasons:
because they feel threatened or uncertain; they are inconvenienced;
their work environment, content or relationships change or if they feel
the change is being imposed on them (Bowman 1986). Lack of information and understanding of what is expected of them, fear of an
increased workload and inadequate resources are often major issues of
concern raised when introducing quality initiatives.

Towell and Harries (1979) recommend that offering information and
support, ensuring effective communication and involving people in
formulating and implementing the activity will help to enhance its
acceptance.

Support from key people
The key people who can help introduce and sustain the initiative should

be identified. These may be the individuals in the organisation who manage the resources, who have the expertise or who are capable of persuading others to accept changes. It is then important to help them see the benefits for themselves, for others and for the organisation.

Plant (1987) believes six activities are central to implementing any change.

(1) Helping individuals or groups face up to change. People need to accept and understand the need to introduce a new idea or way of doing something. If they can see that the new ideas are superior to the old ones, fit in with existing values, are easily understood, relevant to them and can be pretested for success then they are more likely to be accepted (Rogers & Shoemaker 1971).

(2) Communicate like you have never communicated before. Organisational structures and management style are the key to developing effective communication. Structures can be put in place to encourage formal communication upwards, downwards and across an organisation (see Fig. 4.3). Staff also need to understand what their roles and responsibilities are (see Table 4.6 for examples). However, it is the

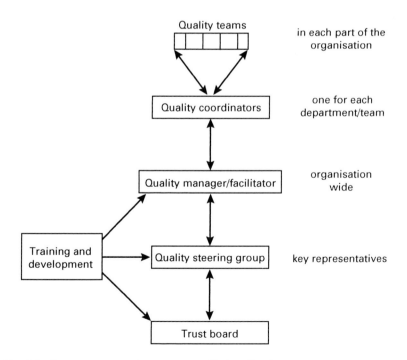

Fig. 4.3 Structures set up to manage quality in a Trust.

Table 4.6   Functions of individuals and groups in the quality strategy.

Teams and departments are responsible for:

- Identifying deficiencies in the quality of their services and making changes to improve.
- Meeting national and local charter standards and quality specifications in contracts.
- Participating in quality monitoring visits and providing information as required by purchasers and users.
- Contributing to the development and implementation of the directorate quality plan.
- Identifying training, support and resources required to meet the quality plan.
- Ensuring a positive image of the Trust is portrayed to patients, visitors and members of the public.

Quality co-ordinators are responsible for working with directorate and department management teams to:

- Ensure the directorate supports the quality strategy.
- Ensure that staff are aware of local and national standards and quality specifications in contracts and ensuring these are achieved.
- Producing a directorate/department quality plan which supports the Trust's plan.
- Identifying training needs of staff to enable them to meet the quality plan.
- Providing reports to the quality steering group.
- Ensuring feedback from consumer surveys is used to improve quality.
- Ensuring action plans resulting from purchaser monitoring visits are implemented.

Quality facilitator has responsibility for:

- Liaising with directorate co-ordinators and the training department to identify and facilitate training.
- Co-ordinating Patient's Charter initiatives.
- Setting up and maintaining systems for monitoring and reporting quality activities.
- Developing, implementing and evaluating specific quality improvement activities across the Trust.
- Support the steering group in its work.

Quality steering group is responsible for:

- Co-ordinating the development, implementation and evaluation of the Trust's quality strategy and quality plan.
- Being proactive in identifying and agreeing quality standards for inclusion in contracts.
- Ensuring information on quality activities from each directorate is included in the annual quality report.
- Receiving purchasers' reports following quality monitoring visits and ensuring appropriate action is taken.
- Identifying and prioritising resources and training required as a result of quality activities.

The **Trust Board** is responsible for:

- Approving and promoting the quality for the Trust.
- Demonstrating commitment to quality by positively promoting the services provided by the Trust.
- Receiving quarterly and annual quality reports.

management style and ethos in the organisation which will help to develop effective relationships in which staff feel sufficiently comfortable and confident to question and contribute to decision making. Developing communication in this way will also help individuals recognise the valuable contribution of others and in turn feel valued themselves.

Communication can be by:

- a regular slot on team brief
- staff newsletter
- specific 'quality' notice boards
- regular slot on departmental meetings
- annual quality report
- formal and informal meetings
- special meetings – workshop, seminars
- formal papers to board and management team meetings
- positive press articles
- networking with key people, e.g. quality co-ordinators.

(3) Gaining energetic commitment to change. Plant (1987) argues that in the short term this involves getting people to focus sharply on the importance of the change for the survival and success of the organisation but in the longer term there should be a system of rewards.

Individuals and groups respond differently to new ideas. There are those who adopt the new approach early and become proactive during the process of developing and introducing the initiative. They are often called opinion leaders or product champions and they can do much to encourage their colleagues to follow suit. They should be identified and encouraged to play a lead in the change.

Similarly change agents are helpful not just in introducing a new idea but also in maintaining the momentum after the initial enthusiasm has waned. Change agents can come from within the organisation but in some situations it may be more helpful to have an external change agent. The advantages of having an internal change agent is that they know the system, understand the values and language used, can identify with the needs and aspiration of the organisation and are a familiar figure (Olson 1979). On the other hand the outsider is independent of the power structure, is in a position to bring in something new and is often seen as an 'expert'.

All activities should be aimed at involving individuals and recognising their contribution as this will increase their interest in, and commitment to, the new idea. Helping them to develop new skills and knowledge required will also assist this process.

(4) Early involvement. One of the most influential factors in introducing successful quality initiatives is the involvement of staff from all relevant groups as early as possible. Failure to involve support staff in a quality initiative in a college of nursing and midwifery in the early stages has proved to be a drawback as the staff felt marginalised and undervalued (Close 1993).

It is possible to involve people at all levels of the organisation (see Fig. 4.3 communication structures). It is important that their involvement is in the main voluntary, as the saying goes, one volunteer is better than ten pressed men. Involvement must however, be supported and an environment which encourages questioning, innovation, problem-solving and critical reflectivity must exist.

(5) Turn perception of threat into opportunities. Organisations which create an environment in which change is seen as a normal occurrence and which encourages staff to be creative and innovative are more likely to encounter less resistance to change.

(6) Avoid over organising. Although it is important to plan changes to introduce new ideas it should be recognised that in reality total control over the change process cannot occur and flexibility is required to take account of the changing circumstances affecting the organisation.

However, an overall framework can be devised which will inform people what contribution they can make and at the same time give them opportunity to develop their own ideas for quality improvement.

Evaluation

An essential part of the strategic process is to evaluate the progress made in developing and implementing the plan. This involves the collection of objective data and then making subjective judgments about it. Although evaluation is the last phase of the cycle, it does not mean that it should only occur at the end.

Formative evaluation is the term used to describe evaluation used as a continuous process throughout the planning cycle. This type of evaluation may indicate that the assessment needs revising or adjustments and modifications need to be made to goals and action plans in the light of information gathered and feedback obtained. Continuous feedback in this way may reveal flaws in the original plan and early corrective intervention may save valuable resources.

Summative evaluation examines the outcomes of the strategic plan against the identified goals. It compares what actually happened with what was planned and answers the question 'How will we know when we have got there?'

The benefits of planned evaluation are that it:

- gives evidence of what has been achieved
- motivates those involved and gives satisfaction when achievements have been recognised
- enables adjustments to be made to meet changing circumstances
- provides a foundation for planned future improvements
- provides evidence of improvements in patient care services or education
- provides evidence that activities are cost effective or of cost benefit.

The evaluation process

(1) Plan the evaluation
Determine the purpose, rationale and scope of the evaluation. There will be a wide range of data that can be collected. To provide information which is manageable in terms of time and effort it is necessary to focus the evaluation. Consider:

- *For whom the evaluation is being done.*
    Who wants the information?
    Who will benefit from it?
- *The purpose of the evaluation.*
    Why is the evaluation being conducted?
- *The scope of the evaluation.*
    Does everything in the plan need to be evaluated?
    What are the key success criteria?
    What resources are there to do the evaluation?

A limited evaluation may be more practical and useful.

(2) Data collection and analysis
The goals and steps identified in the action plan will guide the evaluation and help to identify the tools to be used. The evaluation should combine different approaches and tools to provide both quantitative and qualitative data. It may be necessary to use questionnaires, interviews, discussions, observation and audit of records to collect the information.

(3) Presentation of findings
The essential purpose of the evaluation is to stimulate those involved to reflect on progress and achievements and then decide on action to enhance strengths and diminish weaknesses. A report should be produced which details findings and makes recommendations for further action.

(4) Completing the cycle

Implementing the proposed action and re-evaluation completes the cycle and indicates the centrality of evaluation in the strategic planning process.

Strategic planning ensures a way of anticipating the future and enables the organisation, ward, department or team using it to meet their specific needs. Using this approach encourages staff to work together to use resources effectively and learn from each other with the ultimate aim of providing high quality services to patients.

Discussion points, activities and questions

(1) Consider the factors which influence the development and use of quality activities.
   • To what extent have they had an effect in your area of work?
   • Why do you think they have had such an effect?
   • Could any of these factors help you to develop the quality of services you provide even more?

(2) Are you and the colleagues you work with familiar with the quality specifications in the contracts relating to the area in which you work? If not ask your manager or the person in charge of the contracting process in your organisation if you can see these. It is not possible for you to know whether you are meeting these standards if you don't know what they are.
   When you have seen them discuss with your colleagues and your manager:
   • How well do you think you are meeting them?
   • How are they measured and monitored?
   • Who does this?
   • How often?
   • Is a report produced and do you get to see it?

(3) Are you aware of how contracts are negotiated and who is involved? It will be worth your while to find out how it is done and think of ways in which clinical and teaching staff can be better involved.

(4) Try using the strategic planning cycle in your area of work.

   Phase 1
   • Does the business plan make explicit statements about the quality of services it provides?

- What are the characteristics of your customers?
- What are the characteristics of the staff population working in your area?
- What quality activities are you currently doing?
- What resources and support are available?
- Discuss with your colleagues what sort of management style is operating in the Trust/college? Does this differ to what is in your own area?
- What factors external to your area will influence the development of your quality strategy?

Phase 2

- Try writing goals according to priority of what you want to do over the next year.
- Are they relevant, measurable, precise, understandable, achievable and consistent with the overall objectives of your area?

Phase 3

- How do you make sure the quality of services you provide is good?
- Do you use any tools or frameworks to help you? How effective do you feel they are?
- Have you introduced any changes in the way you work? Was there any resistance from your colleagues? Could you have done it any better?

Phase 4

- To what extent have you evaluated the quality activities you use?
- How do you know they are working?
- Could you do it any better?

References

Alexander, M.F. (1983) *Learning to Nurse. Integrating Theory and Practice.* Churchill Livingstone, Edinburgh.

Balough, R. & Beattie, A. (1988) *Performance Indicators in Nurse Education. Final Report on a Feasibility Study for the ENB.* University of London, Institute of Education, London.

Benton, D. (1994)Performance purchasing. *Nursing Management,* **1**(3), 10–11.

Bowman, M.P. (1986) *Nursing Management and Education: A Conceptual Approach to Change.* Croom Helm, London.

Close, A. (1993) *An examination and evaluation of the change processes involved in developing and implementing a quality assurance strategy in a college of nursing and midwifery.* Unpublished M.Ed dissertation. University of Wales.

Close, A. & MacNeil, M. (1993) Quality strategy in nurse education. *Senior Nurse,* **13**(5), 52–4.

Crosby, P. (1979) *Quality is Free.* McGraw Hill, New York.

DHSS (1972a) *Management Arrangements for the Reorganised Health Service.* (Grey Book.) HMSO, London.

DHSS (1972b) *Report on the Committee on Nursing* (Briggs Report). Cmnd 5115. HMSO, London.

DHSS (1979a) *Patients First.* (Consultative paper on structure and management in the NHS.) DHSS, London.

DHSS (1979b) *Royal Commission on the NHS* (Merrison Report). Cmnd 7615. HMSO, London.

DHSS (1983) *NHS Management Inquiry* (Griffiths). Department of Health and Social Services, London.

DoH (1987) *Promoting Better Health.* Cm 249. HMSO, London.

DoH (1989a) *Caring for People. Community Care in the Next Decade and Beyond.* Cm 849. HMSO, London.

DoH (1989b) *Working for Patients.* Cm 555. HMSO, London.

DoH (1991) *The Patient's Charter.* Department of Health, London.

DoH (1994a) *The Maternity Charter.* Department of Health, London.

DoH (1994b) *The Evolution of Clinical Audit.* Department of Health, London.

DoH (1995) *The Patient's Charter and You.* Department of Health, London.

Donabedian, A. (1966) Evaluating the quality of medical care. *Millbank Fund Quarterly,* **44**(2), 166–206.

ENB (1986) Annual Report 1985/86. English National Board, London.

Fretwell, J.E. (1982) *Ward Teaching and Learning.* Royal College of Nursing, London.

Gott, M. (1983) The preparation of the student for learning in the clinical setting. In: *Research in Nursing,* (ed. B. Davies), pp. 106–128. Croom Helm, London.

Hammer, M. & Champy, J. (1993) *Re-engineering the Corporation: A Manifesto for Business Revolution.* Nicholas Brealey Publishing, London.

Jowett, P. & Rothwell, M. (1988) *Performance Indicators in the Public Sector.* Macmillan Press, Basingstoke.

Juran, J.M. (1988) *Juran on Planning for Quality.* Free Press, New York.

Juran, J.M. (1989) *Juran on Leadership for Quality.* Free Press, New York.

Lang, N. & Clinton, J.F. (1984) Quality assurance – the idea and its development in the United States. In: *Measuring the Quality of Care. Recent Advances in Nursing 10,* (eds L.D. Willis & M.E. Linwood), pp. 69–88. Churchill Livingstone, Edinburgh.

McIver, S. (1993) *Investing in Patient's Representatives.* National Association of Health Authorities and Trusts, Birmingham.

Maxwell, R.J. (1984) Quality assessment in health, *British Medical Journal,* **288**, 1470–2.

Ministry of Health (1947) Working Party on the Recruitment and Training of Nurses (Wood Report). HMSO, London.

NHS (1990) The NHS and Community Care Act 1990. HMSO, London.

NHSE (1994) *Quality and Contracting. Taking the Agenda Forward.* National Health Service Executive Purchasing Unit, London.

NHSE (1995) *Education and Training in the New NHS.* EL(95) 27. March. National Health Service Executive, London.

NHSME (1990a) Working Paper 10 – Education and Training: Interim Guidance Following Consultation. EL(90)MB/94. 30 April 1990. National Health Service Management Executive, London.

NHSME (1990b) Working Paper 10 – Education and Training: Further Guidance. EL(90)/119. 29 June 1990. National Health Service Management Executive, London.

NHSME (1990c) Non-Medical Education and Training; Guidance on Funding Issues. EL(90) 171. 29 August 1990. National Health Service Management Executive, London.

NHSME (1990d) Starting Specifications. A DHA Project Paper. EL(90) 161. August 1990. National Health Service Management Executive, London.

NHSME (1990e) Working Paper 10 – Education and Training: Further Guidance. EL(90) 197. 4 October 1990. National Health Service Management Executive, London.

NHSME (1991) Framework of Audit for Nursing Services. HMSO, London.

Olson, E.M. (1979) Strategies and techniques for the nurse change agent. *Nursing Clinics of North America,* **14**(2), 323–36.

Osborne, S. (1987) A quality circle investigation. *Nursing Times,* 18 February, 73–6.

Øvretveit, J. (1992) *Health Service Quality – An Introduction to Quality Methods for Health Services.* Blackwell Science, Oxford.

Øvretveit, J. (1994) Quality in health service purchasing. *Journal of the Association.* **2**(1), 9–22.

Peters, T.J. & Waterman, R.H. (1982) *In Search of Excellence: Lessons from America's Best-run Companies.* Harper and Row, New York.

Plant, R. (1987) *Managing Change and Making it Stick.* Fontana, London.

RCN (1943) Nursing Reconstruction Committee (Horder Report). Royal College of Nursing, London.

RCN (1987) *Performance Indicators in Nurse Education.* Royal College of Nursing, London.

RCN (1990) *Quality Patient Care: The Dynamic Standard Setting System.* Royal College of Nursing Scutari Projects, Middlesex.

Reid, N. (1985) *Wards in Chancery.* Royal College of Nursing, London.

Rogers, E. & Shoemaker, F. (1971) *Communication of Innovations: A Cross Cultural Report.* The Free Press, New York.

Sale, D. (1990) *Quality Assurance.* Macmillan Education Ltd, Basingstoke.

Towell, D. & Harries, C. (1979) *Innovation in Patient Care.* Croom Helm, London.

UKCC (1992) *Code of Professional Conduct.* United Kingdom Central Council for Nursing, Midwifery and Health Visiting, London.

Walton, M. (1986) *The Deming Management Method.* Putnam, New York.

WHO (1985a) *The Principles of Quality Assurance.* Report on WHO meeting. Euro Report and Studies 94. World Health Organization, Copenhagen.

WHO (1985b) *Targets for Health for All. Targets in Support of the European Regional Strategy for Health for All.* World Health Organization, Copenhagen.

Wilson, C.R.M. (1987) *Hospital Wide Quality Assurance.* University of Toronto Press, Toronto.

Yorke, M. (1991) Performance indicators: Observation on their use in the assurance of course quality. A report for the Council for National Academic Awards. CNAA Project Report 30.

5

Key Concepts in Finance and Information Management

Carol Ward

This complementary chapter is included to provide a much-needed practical overview of concepts relating to the management of finance and information. It starts with a discussion of the functional concepts of budgetary control and provides a helpful explanation of the everyday jargon associated with this area of management, together with an analysis of recurring problems and priorities for practising managers. It then goes on to the more challenging territory of information management, and provides an insight from the author's own substantial experience of implementing information strategies within the British National Health Service (NHS) and industrial settings. Beginning managers and those professionals of all disciplines who are now required to adopt a managerial role will appreciate this concisely written guide through the complexities of both subjects, as will those whose job it is to communicate financial and information strategies to staff in the workplace. Ms Ward has often been described as the answer to the prayers of all those with 'maths phobia'. This chapter is an attempt to condense her wisdom in a readily accessible form for the many readers who have only a limited timescale within which to grasp the essential concepts related to these critical aspects of service management.

Introduction

There have been many changes both within and external to the NHS which have ultimately affected financial management at clinical level. This chapter will therefore begin by identifying these changes in relation to the internal organisational/managerial changes and will then progress to consider the economics of health care. The key concepts of budgeting for clinical managers will then be discussed. The aim is to give the reader an overview of the issues and concepts. There is a further reading section at the end of the chapter should the reader wish to pursue their interests in more detail.

General management

In 1983 a team led by Sir Roy Griffiths produced its report on health service management (DHSS 1983). This report was highly critical at that time and resulted in significant changes to the management of the NHS. The major changes were:

- The appointment of general managers at all levels.
- The introduction of individual performance review and performance related pay.

The overall aims were to ensure accountability for performance, including financial and quality management and to devolve management decision making away from the centre. At the same time management budgeting was introduced and was a precursor to resource management.

Resource management

The major objectives of the resource management initiative (DHSS 1986) were to involve clinicians in the decision-making process, and to improve the use of resources. According to Ham (1991), resource management sought to improve patient care by:

- giving clinical staff a bigger role in the management of resources
- devolving budgetary responsibility to clinical teams within hospitals
- enabling general managers to negotiate levels of activity with these teams
- improving information systems to provide staff with better data about their services.

(The latter is discussed in more detail in the section on information management within this chapter.)

Many UK hospitals, as part of the above, saw the introduction of Clinical Directorates, headed by clinical directors, who in most cases were doctors. Evaluation of the resource management initiative has mainly focused on the improvement of information systems. It is interesting to note however, that very little evaluation appears to have taken place regarding the effectiveness of the Clinical Directorate structure. The implications for clinical staff were obviously a devolution of responsibility for budgets and activity levels. Since the introduction of the NHS reforms (the result of three white papers – *Promoting Better Health* (DoH 1987), *Working for Patients* (DoH 1989b), and *Caring for People* (DoH 1989a), GPs have also been more actively involved in these activities.

The NHS reforms

The reforms resulting from the three white papers detailed above have been said to be the most fundamental since the inception of the NHS in 1948 (Ham 1991). The most significant for this discussion are:

- The separation of purchaser/provider functions resulting in the 'internal market', or managed competition.
- Extension of hospital clinical budgeting (the resource management initiative).
- Creation of NHS Trust hospitals/units, with a long-term objective for all units to become self-governing.
- GP practice budgets for large practices who wish to purchase health care on behalf of their patients.
- Introduction of weighted capitation, as a method of allocation of monies.
- Charges for the use and acquisition of capital.
- Indicative prescribing budgets for GPs.
- Audit of NHS accounts by the Audit Commission.
- Efficiency and effectiveness studies to be carried out by the same Audit Commission.
- Devolution of management, with stronger lines of accountability.

The changes to the health care market originally had many supporters. More recently doubts have been raised (Paton 1995a, 1995b), with some of the original staunch supporters, e.g. Professor Alan Maynard, thought by some to have promoted the idea of GP fund-holding (Maynard 1986), and Professor Chris Ham, originally in favour of the reforms, now becoming more sceptical. Nonetheless the above changes have obvious implications for clinical management, in terms of a decentralisation of responsibility for budgetary control and activity management. Coupled with this increasing accountability, this is a more focused approach to measuring efficiency and effectiveness of care. In addition the economics of health care are also changing.

Economics and health care

There is continuing debate relating to expenditure on health, with differences of opinion as to whether this has increased or decreased (in real terms), dependent on which side of the political fence one sits. According to Begg *et al.* (1994), real expenditure (i.e. inflation adjusted) between 1981 and 1991 actually increased by 30 per cent. The latter author also states however, that the public's perception is that there have been substantial cutbacks in health care funding.

If expenditure has actually increased, therefore, why is there such a widely held perception? Spending on health care has increased at the same rate as the rest of national output. There are, however, other factors which are increasing the pressure on health care resources – the increasing numbers of elderly people and advances in medical technology are examples. In reality, if we are to meet these needs then expenditure as a percentage of output will need to increase. Alternatively, greater debate on health care rationing will need to take place (Spinks 1994).

Against this background of internal managerial changes and external pressures, clinical managers are now expected to have greater involvement in managing resources, at a time when conflicts are greater than ever. The key concepts relating to budgeting will therefore now be discussed.

Key concepts of budgeting

A definition of a budget given by Harrison (p. 113) in 1989 is:

'A financial or quantitative statement, prepared in advance of a period of time, reflecting the agreed policies and strategies necessary to meet objectives.'

The majority of us manage a personal budget – some better than others! Organisational budgets do, however, have more specific objectives (Taylor 1992) which are outlined below:

- *As a process to prioritise.* The definition of potential planned budgets enables the overall organisation to decide where the priorities must be. Unfortunately this usually means that not all budget-holders' expectations are met.
- *To secure resources for the organisation.* Costing of activity and hence potential budgetary requirements must be identified in order to present a case to purchasers when agreeing contractual activity and cost.
- *To communicate, co-ordinate and control activities within the organisation.* Formal budget plans are the mechanisms by which overall plans are communicated to middle managers, with responsi-

bility delegated accordingly. In order to motivate the latter and ensure goal congruence, it is vital that managers are involved in the planning and budget setting stages. Co-ordination between departments is vital, particularly where a number of departments are involved in the same project, e.g. a waiting list initiative. Control of activities, and hence expenditure, is probably the element of budgeting that most affects clinical managers. This will be discussed later in terms of costing and charging, monitoring expenditure, and activity and expenditure.

- *Performance measurement.* Budgetary control is still the primary measure of performance for operational managers. This is often very frustrating for clinical managers who may feel that other measures should be utilised.

Budgetary planning/preparation

There are two main approaches to preparing a budget: *incremental* and *zero-based budgeting.*

The term *incremental* is used where the previous year's budget is adjusted to take into account changes brought about by:

- inflation
- changes in activity levels
- cost improvement programmes
- service developments.

Unfortunately even if any of the above occur, it does not always mean that changes are made to the planned budget. For example, activity levels may increase without any subsequent increase in finance. The outcome therefore is a significant cost improvement programme, or changes in other aspects of service performance, such as quality or flexibility. Clinical managers must therefore have an understanding of key budgetary concepts and must become confidently involved in the planning process.

Zero-based budgeting is the exact opposite of incremental budgeting in that it assumes no previous activity or expenditure. This is not often used in the health service, apart from when undertaking value for money studies or setting up a totally new service. With the latter however, this is often still not zero-based in its truest form in that previous information regarding costs may be utilised. Clinical managers are often asked to get involved in the costing or recharging of their service, therefore an understanding of the key terms must be gained.

Costing and charging

There are numerous types of costs which are allocated to cost centres. These are often described in various ways (for a more detailed account please refer to one of the management accounting texts referred to in the bibliography provided). For the purposes of this chapter the following will be discussed:

- cost categories
- components of costs – direct/indirect and overheads, and fixed and variable.

Cost categories
There are various classifications, the most simple being between staff and non-staff costs. Currently however, this is becoming more sophisticated, with costs relating specifically to items of expenditure/service, examples of which (taken from Greenhalgh 1991) are:

- basic staff costs
- special duty payments
- overtime
- salary related costs (employees' National Insurance, superannuation – sometimes referred to as on-costs)
- drugs/dressings
- laundry
- CSSD
- catering
- supplies
- stationery and equipment

The allocation and categorisation of these costs will be dependent on local definitions, accounting systems and administrative policies. Although there are numerous categories, a typical ward budget consists of nearly 90 per cent expenditure on staff. In the author's experience however, when asked to consider cost improvement programmes at ward level, clinical staff often focus on the non-staff budgets such as supplies. Effective utilisation of staff as a resource is obviously a key element of a clinical manager's responsibility in budgetary control.

Components of costs

(1) Direct/indirect and overheads
Direct costs are those costs which can be attributed directly to that service, and hence should be controlled by the budget holder, examples being staffing costs, or supplies needed for patients in that area.

Indirect costs are usually costs of services provided by other departments and are therefore controlled by another budget holder – an example of which may be portering or physiotherapy. In order to maintain some control, some units have introduced service level agreements or cross charging. In reality the latter is often very expensive to set up and maintain when compared to the benefits incurred.

Overheads are usually the costs which are controlled by the organisation, i.e. those that are not easy to apportion (divide out). Examples of these would be maintenance and car parking.

As accounting systems become more sophisticated, cross charging and apportionment may become more common. This may still have its frustrations in that managers may have very little control in the ongoing monitoring once targets have been agreed.

(2) Fixed/variable

Fixed costs are the components of a service which are fixed and which do not alter with the level of activity – an example of which may be the cost of the building in which activity takes place, or equipment required.

Variable costs are costs which fluctuate with demand, for example staffing or supplies. The distinction however, is not always crystal clear, some costs can be semi-fixed or semi-variable. As activity significantly increases additional equipment may be required – an example of what is meant by the term *semi-fixed*.

On a ward a core number of staff are required to open even a limited number of beds. As activity increases however, this number of staff does not usually need to increase per patient, but at a certain increase in number of patients treated, additional staff would be required. This is often referred to as stepped costs, and is an example of what is meant by the term *semi-variable*.

Monitoring expenditure

Also referred to as *variance analysis*, this requires the manager to monitor the ongoing expenditure against the original planned budget. Over or underspends must be investigated. Investigation usually starts by assessing the financial statement itself. Are there any data errors? For example, have all employees been coded to the correct cost centre? Further investigation may require the analysis of pay roll data, establishing whether any changes in activity have occurred, and/or whether there have been excessive amounts of sickness/maternity leave which required the utilisation of agency staff. Apart from data errors, most managers should be able to identify very quickly why a variance has occurred. Indeed a proactive manager should be highlighting in advance whether budgetary variances are likely to occur.

Activity and expenditure

The author has often heard clinical staff state that they do not feel they manage a budget if they are not required to undertake variance analysis. In reality the budget is 'managed' by constantly managing the resources, e.g. by effective rostering, monitoring of sickness, monitoring of activity and changes in practice. Most clinical managers therefore manage a budget even if it is their manager who is held responsible and who undertakes variance analysis. The key to managing this successfully is the level of involvement in the decision-making process and the amount of control held.

In many industries *activity based costing* (ABC) has been introduced. This involves the matching of activity to costs. In the NHS this was referred to as management budgeting in some hospitals in the 1980s, and attempts were made to link costs to activity. Unfortunately ABC requires flexible budgets and the NHS is a cash limited service. In theory, contracting was supposed to enable this process, i.e. the more activity, the more money should be paid. In reality purchasers are also cash limited, therefore it is unlikely that true flexible budgeting will ever occur. Some departments are able to operate on this basis such as Central Sterile Supply Departments. Most clinical services however, find it very difficult to restrain activity. Attempts are now being made to identify the extent of this problem by the introduction of service level agreements between departments such as physiotherapy and occupational therapy services. There are obvious problems, however, when accident and emergency departments are funded for a certain level of activity. If they overperform does an increased budget always follow, or should rationing of the service take place? If so how would the latter be managed? These are obviously the potential frustrations and conflicts for clinical managers.

Performance measurement

Performance measurement in the NHS has tended to focus on financial and activity-based measures. Until recently this was mainly directed at senior and middle management, however many organisations are introducing this form of measurement to clinical staff. A news item in the *Health Service Journal* (Butler 1995), states that many Trusts are linking pay offers to performance, linked to the numbers of patients treated and relative success in meeting overall Trust financial targets.

Many authors state that, in isolation, measuring these types of financial and activity targets is inappropriate, and that attention should also be focused on multiple dimensions of performance (Bromwich & Bhimani 1989; Fitzgerald *et al.* 1991). Other dimensions often relate to the quality of service provided which has been discussed by Ann Close in Chapter 4. Until all dimensions of performance are measured, therefore, clinical managers may suffer conflict and frustration if their performance is measured mainly on financial indicators.

To conclude, this section has given an overview of financial management for clinical managers. External and internal pressures have resulted in increasing decentralised responsibility for activity and budgetary management. There is also increasing pressure to measure the efficiency and effectiveness of services. It is vital therefore that all clinical managers must be knowledgeably and actively involved in all aspects of budgetary management. This section was intended to 'whet the appetite' of the reader, and to help them become more comfortable with financial management jargon. A bibliography is given at the end of this chapter to facilitate further study of this demanding and complex area of management study.

Information Management: An Introduction

The original brief for this section was to consider the concepts and application of information technology (IT) for health care. The astute amongst you will note that this has now been changed to discuss information systems, rather than IT in isolation. This is a deliberate attempt on my part to enable the reader to think broadly in terms of utilising information to enhance the clinical process, in addition to promoting more efficient data for operational management, contracting and costing.

A distinction must therefore be drawn between information systems and information technology. According to Earl (1989) information systems are the *what* of utilising information. That is, what information is required to enable the management of the service. Information technology is the *how*. That is, how can technology be applied to improve information systems. It must, therefore, be acknowledged from the beginning that information systems, both formal and informal, need not be computerised.

In American industry for example, where in theory the use of IT is more advanced, McKinnon and Burns (1992), point out that managers still get two-thirds of their information from face-to-face or telephone conversations. The remaining third comes from documents, most of which were not available on their computer systems.

In health care however, as Barry and Gibbons (1990) state, one only has to consider the massive amount of information that nurses and other professionals manage to appreciate that we need adequate systems to process that data in order to improve the effectiveness of care. To identify appropriate information systems we must therefore consider how people use information, not how people use machines (Davenport 1994).

This section will therefore consider how best we can define what information systems are required in the delivery of health care. Before we can consider how this can be approached it is useful, however, to consider the historical background to information management in the NHS.

Historical background

In 1979 the Royal Commission highlighted the inadequacy of information at that time:

'The information available to assist decision makers in the NHS leaves much to be desired. Relevant information may not be available at all, or in the wrong form. Information that is produced is often too late to assist decisions, or may be of dubious accuracy'.

(DHSS 1979 cited in Greenhalgh 1993)

Since that time there have been a number of developments in information management in the NHS, partly as a result of changes in its overall management. Examples of these developments will be discussed briefly below.

(1) The Korner reports (DHSS 1982–1984)

These reports were produced in an attempt to improve information management in the NHS. The key concept resulting from this was the introduction of *minimum data sets* (MDS). These were intended to improve the standardisation of definitions of data across the country. The philosophy of data collection was based on the belief that the most effective way of collecting data was at operational level. This collection was therefore often carried out by clinical staff, e.g. physiotherapists, community nurses, etc. At that time many manual and computerised systems were of a poor quality and those collecting the data often had very little feedback. The recommendations have therefore been criticised on many counts (Greenhalgh 1993). It must be remembered, however, that the introduction of MDS was a necessary precursor to raising awareness of the importance of information in the management of health care.

During this stage the majority of units also began to introduce *patient administration systems* (PAS), which were to support operational management. At this stage however, these were mainly centralised systems which were not utilised directly by clinical staff.

(2) Resource management

The major objectives of the resource management initiative (DHSS 1986) were to involve clinicians in the decision-making process and to improve the use of resources. In order to achieve this, there were two key elements: *organisation and development,* and the introduction of *patient based information systems.*

During the late 1980s and early 1990s there was therefore, a drive to introduce specific core information systems, these being:

- patient administration systems (PAS)
- case mix management systems (CMMS)
- clinical information/clinical workstations for medical audit
- nursing information systems.

In addition, hospitals implementing resource management were expected to establish at least two additional departmental feeder systems (i.e. systems that would feed information into the CMMS), for example in theatres, pathology, x-ray and pharmacy. Monies were allocated via regional resource management teams to support these initiatives. Whereas numerous successive innovations have undoubtedly occurred (Cross 1994), there have also been a number of reported disasters (Chadda 1994). In addition the evaluation of clinical systems, such as nursing information systems, did not meet the original expectations of implementation (Audit Commission 1992). This will be discussed later when considering information requirements.

(3) NHS reforms/the internal market

Following the white paper *Working for Patients* (DoH 1989b), the creation of the internal market – i.e. the division into purchasers of health care (health authorities and GPs), and providers of care (hospitals, community services and so on) – has resulted in an even greater need for speedy, accurate, accessible information across all areas of health care management. For example, to enable costing and charging of services; medical and clinical audit; monitoring of health care provision and outcomes, and monitoring of consequent purchaser quality standards.

Additional pressures for better information have resulted from the introduction of Patient's Charter Standards (DoH 1991, 1995), the subsequent need to monitor performance, and the white paper *Caring for People* (DoH 1989a) all of which have resulted in the need to improve information flows; not only within organisations, but with external customers/providers, for example hospital to general practitioner, and vice versa. Unfortunately however, many organisations' information systems were inadequate to cope with significant changes experienced by the new NHS.

In an attempt to improve information management *An Information Management and Technology Strategy for the NHS in England* (NHS Management Executive (NHSME 1992)) was produced in 1992.

(4) Information management and technology (IM&T) strategy

There are certain key principles within the strategy:

- Non repetitiveness of data, i.e. all individuals should have one NHS number.
- Operational data should be utilised so that information should be collected where care is delivered.

- Security and confidentiality of information is essential, therefore although information should be accessible and shared across the NHS via a network of computers, standards should be in place to maintain these basic principles of health care.

There are therefore a number of national projects currently under way to achieve the above. Information regarding these can be found in the various booklets and briefing notes produced by the NHSME as part of the IM&T (see the bibliography below). Examples of the projects:

- Hospital Information Support Systems (HISS).
- Community Information Systems for Providers (CISP).
- Developing Information Systems for Purchasers (DISP).
- A new format NHS number.
- A national thesaurus of coded clinical terms and groupings.
- NHS wide 'networking'.
- Framework for Security and Confidentiality.

There is also a drive within the strategy to involve users in defining information requirements. In my experience this is not always as easy as it appears. For the last three years the author has been leading the development of a nursing information strategy, as part of an acute hospital-wide information strategy. What transpired was that clinical staff had seldom reflected constructively on what information was required to manage clinical care; for example what elements needed to be computerised, and had certainly not considered the wider professional and organisational implications of corporate information requirements.

I will therefore consider two models which may be used to identify information system requirements, i.e. *what* information is required, and *how* information technology may, or may not, now assist in the process.

Due to my own professional background this will be considered in the context of an acute hospital setting. However, the principles can apply in any sector, as the models themselves originated in the industrial setting and not health care.

Identifying information requirements

A simple model for defining information requirements is shown in Fig. 5.1. This is based on a model developed by Nolan in 1979. As can be seen this is a traditional hierarchical model which divides activity, and hence information requirements, into:

- strategic planning systems
- management control systems
- operational/process control systems.

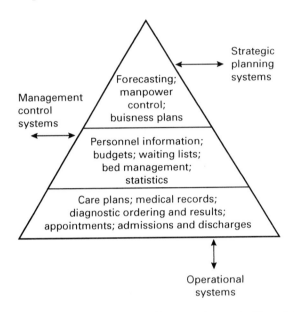

Fig. 5.1 Planning, control and operational systems in a typical hospital setting – a traditional hierarchical application model based on Anthony's (1965) structuring of management activities. Adapted, with permission of John Wiley & Sons Ltd, from *Strategic Planning for Information Systems* by John Ward *et al.* (1993).

Examples have been given within the model itself as to how this may be applied to health care. This model has been criticised within the IT world, mainly for its simplicity (King & Kraemer 1984). King and Kraemer point out however, that it is this same simplicity which represented the key to its popularity, making it easy to understand by practitioners of various and diverse backgrounds.

For this reason the author believes that this may be a useful starting point when considering information requirements in health care. It is useful to ensure that these are assessed not only in relation to the clinical management of care, but also in relation to the management of resources. The management/control and strategic aspects of this model will be returned to later.

When considering the process of health care however, a more useful model may be that shown in Fig. 5.2. Known as the 'value added model' identified by Michael E. Porter in 1985, this has since been utilised as a useful framework for identifying information requirements in an organisation (Ward *et al.* 1993).

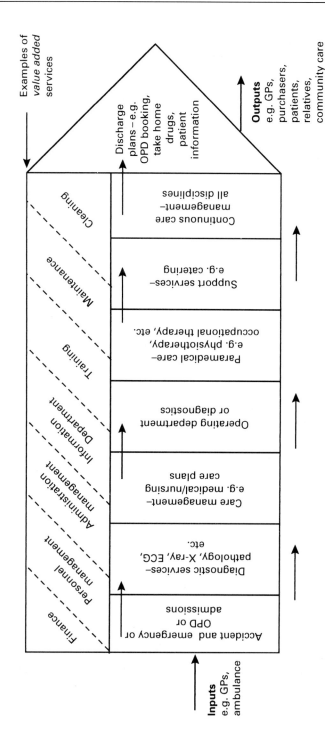

Fig. 5.2 The process of Health Care in a Hospital Setting. Adapted, with permission of The Free Press, an imprint of Simon & Schuster, from *Competitive Advantage: Creating and Sustaining Superior Performance* by Michael E. Porter. Copyright © 1985 by Michael E. Porter.

As can be seen from the examples given, the bottom of the model equates to the process of care. An advantage of this type of approach is that it takes into account inputs and outputs – in this example information flows between purchasers of health care and community care, in addition to the receivers of care (the patient). In addition, it enables a focused approach to information flows *around* the process of care, rather than individual functions. Some of the criticisms of earlier information systems were that they focused on individual departments, e.g. x-ray, accident and emergency, or functional professional groups such as nursing. This often resulted in fragmented approaches to the use of IT, which did not ultimately enhance patient care.

The upper part of the model are what Porter described as *value added* services, that is services which add value to the overall process. The need for increasing information relating to these areas will be dependent on how critical these are to the overall service. An example of this would be the need for effective personnel management in terms of recruitment and retention, training, health and safety, i.e. a service which would directly affect the welfare of staff, and hence indirectly the process of care delivery.

When reviewing the potential of HISS or CISP therefore, Porter's model would appear to enable a focus on the information requirements of multidisciplinary care focused around patient care delivery.

For the purpose of illustration, I will now offer examples of information flows across a hospital, in relation to the above model, and demonstrate how information technology may or may not assist in this process.

Initial contact

According to the above model, this is the *input* stage of care. This may be for example, correspondence from GPs, or initial reception at accident and emergency departments. Currently this initial stage is mainly in the form of manual data. For example a GP may refer a patient to a particular consultant, a letter is sent, coding takes place, a medical record is either prepared or found and an appointment made. The patient may then need to attend follow-up appointments given for diagnostic tests, before another appointment for potential diagnosis and any necessary admission date.

The use of appropriate technology could drastically improve the above process. An effective PAS system with links to x-ray, pathology and other departments, in addition to direct access for GPs could enable direct ordering of diagnostic tests by GPs. In addition an out-patients appointment could be booked directly by the GP's receptionist.

On arrival at clinic, results would then be available for reference, and if the patient needed to be admitted the consultant should then be able to provisionally book a bed on the bed management system.

Obviously this type of immediate access for GPs would require changes to operational processes. It must also be recognised that improvements in information flows do not solve all problems, notably bed availability, however effective management is dependent on fast information flows.

In patient care

The above is only one example of the initial phase of hospital care. Once admitted there are numerous examples of information flows including:

- patient records
- order communications and reporting systems
- verbal handovers
- multidisciplinary protocols
- patient/relative information
- bed management
- discharge planning
- community links

A brief discussion of each will now follow.

Patient records

At the time of writing there are a number of Trusts involved in piloting the electronic patient record (EPR) project (Anon 1994). The aim is to computerise all aspects of patient records. It is obviously too early to discuss this in detail, however one of the pilot sites (Burton hospital) has had some success in developing computerised records, within its HISS system. Unfortunately this success does not appear to be commonplace. During the resource management era, millions of pounds were spent on nursing information systems. The Audit Commission in 1992 found numerous problems had occurred in the introduction of computerised nursing care plans. These are summarised below:

- Time and effort involved – not only in developing the original system, but in ensuring that care actually delivered is recorded.
- Care plans were difficult to use – these were often too long, required numerous print-outs, therefore resulting in increasing amounts of paper records.
- Computer terminals taking much needed nurses away from the bedside.

- Care plans were often not individualised. Where this was done, this was often manually, therefore that data were not necessarily retained.
- It was more difficult to involve the patient; although some areas had tried to introduce bedside or hand-held terminals, this still did not enable patient participation to take place.
- Restricted learning and opportunities for reflective practice – there were some nurses who felt that computerised care plans discouraged nurses from giving adequate thought to appropriate care planning.
- Where care plans were used for workload assessment, the plans were often task lists, which again detracted from individualised care.

Before computerising records we must therefore establish the true purpose of doing so and assess whether this will improve patient care. There is obviously scope to utilise IT in assisting in the process, for example by printing records containing patient details thereby preventing duplication of effort. Word processor facilities could be useful to enable localised core care plans to be developed. Order communication systems (see below) may also enable faster information flows between departments and professional groups with regard to the individual patient. Where care is dynamic and tailored to the individual patient, it has yet to be seen whether the fully integrated EPR systems will be successful.

Systems order communication and reporting systems
Order communication systems (OCS) are systems which transfer requests and associated results between support departments and wards. These are more usually associated with pathology, radiology and pharmacy. At Burton however, where a HISS is established, support services such as physiotherapy, occupational therapy and so on are linked into the system.

There would appear to be obvious benefits to such systems, for example enabling speedier information flows relating directly to patient care and potential development of clinical protocols. What must be acknowledged when considering systems such as OCS however, is the need for discussion between various professional groups regarding potential changes to current operational processes. For example, who will order routine blood tests and will these be built into protocols of care?

Verbal handovers
This form of information exchange is still common and extensively used within most hospitals. In a recent audit carried out at my own hospital, it was found that when busy, nurses often stated that they did not have

time to update care plans. However it was only on very rare occasions that the 'handover' did not take place. This form of data exchange is not often recorded and therefore has its limitations in promoting continuity of care and in recording patient care for future reference.

One suggestion put forward by the Audit Commission (1992), was that recording of care may be speeded up if nurses were provided with dictation facilities and secretarial support. It will be interesting to see whether any hospitals put this suggestion into practice! One development in IT which may assist in the process is *speech to text*. By speaking into a microphone this can be translated into a typed record. Again, whether hospitals will be able to invest in this type of technology for the foreseeable future is doubtful. It would appear that verbal handovers will continue. It follows that whatever methods are employed in the longer term more emphasis must be placed on the recording of care as this is integral to the process of care delivery (NHSME 1991).

Multidisciplinary protocols
With the current drive towards clinical audit (DoH 1994), there is a need to develop multidisciplinary protocols. As stated above, these may usefully enable aspects of care to be undertaken automatically and hence enable faster information flows. They may also be useful for retrospective audit studies of care.

The issues relating to computerised care plans are also pertinent to protocols. In my view, health care professionals must beware of totally standardising care. True protocols must also involve all health care professionals and not just be based on medical directives.

Patient/relative information
Although numerous information booklets are now produced, the majority of information flows still appear to be verbal. There is obvious potential in exploring the use of technology to assist in this process. This could take the simple form of audio-visual aids such as explanatory cassettes and videos. Long term however, there may be scope for the use of interactive multimedia. In addition it may not be too many years before patients can, via a network, have access to relevant and user friendly health care information. Currently however, there is still a need to identify how best we can support verbal information with better alternatives.

Bed management
Many PAS systems now have the capacity to enable allocation of beds. Advocates of these systems state that this enables quicker admission from accident and emergency departments. Any information system is

dependent on staff inputting timely data. If clinical staff do not immediately input that a patient has been discharged, that bed will still be considered as occupied. This is one very clear example as to how clinical staff must have adequate training and an allegiance towards corporate philosophy and goals for information systems to realise their potential in health care.

Discharge planning and community links
Currently often manual discharge planning could be improved by applied technology. Appointments could be made, prescribed medication ordered, ambulances booked, community services contacted, and GP letters transferred via a HISS and a link to community services. There is therefore I would argue, enormous potential for IT to improve this process.

Operational and strategic management

Utilising Nolan's (1979) earlier model, in addition to the above examples of information flows in the process of care, it is necessary to consider *operational management*, those activities Porter (1985) would describe as *adding value*. Examples of these are:

- personnel systems
- financial management
- quality management
- communication
- contracting/forecasting/patient scheduling

and these are discussed briefly below.

Personnel systems

Information relating to personnel management includes staff records, sickness and absence, and training details. A strategic decision needs to be made as to what information is more easily stored in a computer, remembering the issues of: who will input the data, who will need access to that information, and therefore at what level that information should ideally be held.

Rostering systems could be considered as personnel or financial information systems. Automated systems have not been successful to date (Audit Commission 1992). Problems include not actually saving nurses' time and a general lack of flexibility. The main benefits have been seen by managers rather than ward staff. If linked to a financial system, costing of nursing care can take place. Problems have arisen, however, in the need to constantly update and incorporate planned off-duties.

There is potential to record attendance at ward/departmental level to improve the effectiveness of payroll systems and costing of care. In my view this again could be enhanced with the assistance of IT.

Financial management

All hospitals have financial information systems, of which some are more sophisticated than others. There are also variances relating to whether financial information is centralised or decentralised. Examples of financial information flows for health care professionals are dependent on the extent to which the staff are involved in budgetary control and costing of activity. On initial consideration most wards/departments may feel that they require instant access to financial data. The concept of *added value* therefore needs to be considered here. It may be just as useful to have a monthly statement of activity and expenditure.

Numerous hospitals have implemented workload systems in an attempt to improve forecasting, scheduling and costing. Concerns have been expressed, however, as to the actual benefits incurred (Audit Commission 1992; Jenkins-Clarke 1992).

Quality management

Various types of information are required in relation to quality. This may include incident rates of complaints, wound care, infection rates and so on; care protocols, information for clinical auditing, Patient's Charter information and various other indicators specified within the contracting process. It would appear that IT may assist in this type of data collection and monitoring. Before considering expenditure on software however, consideration must be given to the fact that quality management is dynamic, therefore any packages must be sufficiently flexible and adaptable.

Communication systems

Various communication systems currently exist. These include briefings, internal memorandums, letters, telephone calls, newsletters, ward/departmental meetings. Information flows can be speeded up by facilities such as electronic-mail (e-mail), however it must be remembered that this still takes time to read and/or download!

Contracting/forecasting/scheduling

There are both operational and strategic elements to the above. As stated earlier, accurate information is vital to enable the contracting process to be effective. The potential is also there to forecast trends relating to health care, and hence enable more effective scheduling. Those wishing to read further should consider *Using Information in Contracting* (Greenhalgh 1993).

Conclusion

To summarise and conclude: there have been numerous changes in the NHS which have directly affected the delivery and management of care. Consideration of information requirements is therefore more important than ever. Two established models in strategic planning for information systems have been utilised here in order to demonstrate the various levels and processes which need to be considered when identifying information requirements in an acute hospital setting.

Health care is regrettably too complex to discuss all areas. The examples given were intended to illustrate how information is an essential part of the care process and its management. Time must be given to consider future information flows. Technology will give opportunities to improve care, but a note of caution is necessary here. IT cannot be seen as a panacea to all communication problems. As stated earlier, there is a need to consider *what* information is required and then *how* technology can improve information flows. This assessment also gives the opportunity to review and change actual processes involved.

We need to consider how people use *information* rather than how they use technology. Operational and clinical staff must therefore be fully involved in debates about information flows and the future of information technology and effective provision of health care.

References

Anon (1994) News item: Two Trusts will lead NHS into computer age. *Health Service Journal*, **104**(5428), 7.

Audit Commission (1992) *Caring Systems: A Handbook for Nursing and Project Managers. HMSO, London.*

Barry, C.T. & Gibbons, L.K. (1990) Information systems technology: barriers and challenges to implementation, *Journal of Nursing Administration*, **20**(2), 40–42.

Begg, D., Fischer, S. & Dornbusch, R. (1994) *Economics*, 4th edn. McGraw-Hill, England.

Bromwich, M. & Bhimani, A. (1989) *Management Accounting: Evolution Not Revolution.* Chartered Institute of Management Accountants, London.

Butler, P. (1995) News item. *Health Service Journal*, **105**(5448), 7.

Chadda, D. (1994) News item. West Midlands health chiefs wasted millions on computer project. *Health Service Journal*, **104**(5387), 7.

Cross, M. (1994) The HISS that got away. *Health Service Journal*, **104**(5430), 8–9.

Davenport, T.H. (1994) Saving IT's soul: human centred information management. *Harvard Business Review*, Mar–Apr, 119–31.

DHSS (1979) *Report of the Royal Commission of the NHS.* Cmm 7615. HMSO, London.

DHSS (1982–1984) Steering Group on Health Services Information. Chaired By E. Korner. Six reports to the Secretary of State. HMSO, London.

DHSS (1983) *NHS Management Inquiry – Chaired by Roy Griffiths.* HMSO, London.

DHSS (1986) *Health Services Management: Resource Management in Health Authorities (Management Budgeting).* HN(86)34. HMSO, London.

DoH (1987) *Promoting Better Health.* Cm 249. HMSO, London.

DoH (1989a) *Caring for People: Community Care in the Next Decade and Beyond.* Cm 849. HMSO, London.

DoH (1989b) *Working for Patients.* Cm 555. HMSO, London.

DoH (1991) *The Patient's Charter.* HMSO, London.

DoH (1994) *NHS Executive: Improving the Effectiveness of the NHS.* (94) 74. Department of Health, London.

DoH (1995) *The Patient's Charter and You.* HMSO, London.

Earl, M.J. (1989) *Management Strategies for Information Technology.* Prentice Hall, Hemel Hempstead.

Fitzgerald, L., Johnson, R., Brignall, S., *et al.* (1991) *Performance Measurement in Service Business.* Chartered Institute of Management Accountants, London.

Greenhalgh and Co. Ltd (1991) in conjunction with a five regional consortium. Financial management. In: *Using Information in Managing the Nursing Resource.* Greenhalgh and Co. Ltd, Macclesfield.

Greenhalgh and Co. Ltd (1993) in conjunction with a five regional consortium. *Using Information in Contracting – Setting the Context.* HMSO, London.

Griffiths, R. (1983) *NHS Management Enquiry.* DHSS, London.

Ham, C. (1991) *The New National Health Service.* Radcliffe Medical Press, Oxford.

Harrison, J. (1989) *Finance for the Non-financial Manager.* Harper Collins, London.

Jenkins-Clarke, S. (1992) *Measuring Nursing Workload: A Cautionary Tale.* Centre for Health Economics, University of York, York.

King, J.L. & Kraemer, K.L. (1994) Evolution and organisational information systems: an assessment of Nolan's stage model. *Communications of ACM*, **27**, 5 (May).

King, W.R. (1984) Evolution and organisational information systems: an assessment of Nolan's stage model. *Communications of ACM*, 27 May, 5. Cited in Ward, J., Griffiths, P. & Whitmore, P. (1993). John Wiley & Sons, Chichester.

McKinnon, S.M. & Burns, W.J. (1992) *The Information Mosaic.* Harvard School Press, Boston.

Maynard, A. (1986) Performance incentives. In: *Health, Education and General Practice,* (ed. G. Teeling Smith). Office of Health Economics, London.

NHSME (1991) *Keeping the Record Straight.* National Health Service Management Executive, HMSO, London.

NHSME (1992) *An Information Management and Technology Strategy for the NHS in England.* National Health Service Management Executive, HMSO, London.

Nolan, R.L. (1979) Managing the crises in data processing, *Harvard Business Review,* Mar–Apr.

Paton, C. (1995a) Present dangers and future threats; some perverse incentives in the NHS, *British Medical Journal,* **310**(6989), 1245–8.

Paton, C. (1995b) Change is as good as a rest, *Health Service Journal,* **105**(5460), 24–5.

Porter, M.E. (1985) *Competitive Advantage: Creating and Sustaining Superior Performance.* Free Press, New York.

Spinks, M. (1994) Widening the rationing debate, *Nursing Times,* **90**(34), 24–30.

Taylor, N. (1992) *Budgeting Skills: A Guide for Nurse Managers.* Quay Publishing, Lancaster.

Ward, J., Griffiths, P. & Whitmore, P. (1993) *Strategic Planning for Information Systems.* John Wiley & Sons, Chichester.

Suggested further reading

General Economics

Begg, D., Fischer, S. & Dornbusch, R. (1994) *Economics,* 4th edn. McGraw-Hill, England.

Nellis, J.G. & Parker, D. (1990) *The Essence of the Economy.* Prentice Hall, Hemel Hempstead.

Economics and health care

Appleby, J. (1992) *Financing Health Care in the 1990s.* Open University Press, Buckingham.

Mooney, G. (1992) *Economics, Medicine and Health Care,* 2nd edn. Harvester Wheatsheaf, London.

Spinks, M. (1994) Widening the rationing debate. *Nursing Times,* **90**(34), 24–30.

Health care markets

Butler J. (1992) *Patients, Policies and Politics: Before and After 'Working for Patients'.* Open University Press, Buckingham.

Ham, C. (1991) *The New National Health Service.* Radcliffe Medical Press, Oxford.

Taylor-Goodby, P. & Lawson, R. (1993) *Markets and Managers: New Issues in the Delivery of Welfare.* Open University Press, Buckingham.

Budgeting

Atrill, P. & McLaney, E. (1994) *Management Accounting: An Active Learning Approach.* Blackwell Business, Oxford.

Greenhalgh and Co. Ltd. (1991) in conjunction with a five regional consortium. Financial Management. In: *Using Information in Managing the Nursing Resource.* Greenhalgh and Co. Ltd, Macclesfield.

Harrison, J. (1989) *Finance for the Non-financial Manager.* Harper Collins, London.

Jones, A. & McDonnell, U. (1993) *Managing the Clinical Resource.* Baillière Tindall, London.

Lucey, T. (1988) *Management Accounting,* 2nd edn. DP Publications, London.

Pelfrey, S. (1990) Cost categories, behaviour patterns and break-even analysis. *Journal of Nursing Administration,* **20**(12), 10–14.

Shafer, W. (1991) Managing a budget at ward level. *Professional Nurse,* **6**(11), 677–80.

Taylor, N. (1992) *Budgeting Skills: A Guide for Nurse Managers.* Quay Publishing, Lancaster.

Information management

Greenhalgh and Co. Ltd (1991) in conjunction with a five regional consortium. *Using Information in Managing the Nursing Resource.* HMSO, London.

Greenhalgh and Co Ltd (1993) in conjunction with a five regional consortium. *Using Information in Contracting – PG 401 – Setting the Context.* HMSO, London.

NHSME (1992) *An Information Management and Technology Strategy for the NHS in England.* National Health Service Management Executive, London. Published as 43 separate booklets and 43 briefing notes including:

IM & T Strategy Overview

A View for General Medical Practitioners.

A View for Community Nurses.

A View for Hospital Nurses.

A View for Hospital Doctors.

HISS: Pulling IT Together in Hospitals.

HISS: Implications of Implementation.

A New Format NHS Number.

What are Read Codes?

A National Thesaurus of Clinical Terms in Read Codes.

Towards a Language for Health.

Towards NHS Wide Networking.

Introducing ICD10.

Information Security and You.
Realising the Benefits of HISS.
IM & T Training.

Part III

EDUCATION AND TRAINING IN HEALTH CARE

6
A Critique of Alternative Pathways in Professional and Vocational Education

Terry Hyland

This chapter is a powerful and authoritative critique of recent policy developments in education and training in health care. It addresses questions facing education providers and purchasers, and directly challenges some of the common assumptions held by employers, educationalists and human resource developers. For example, is training a form of social control? Are the present competence-based educational initiatives too limited in scope to address the complexities of future health care provision and management? Does increasing centralisation of control over the education system carry implications for future educational and workforce planning, and the subsequent creation of opportunities for professional and vocational development? What are the potentially contentious issues confronting policy-makers and funding agencies, and what challenges must service and education managers therefore rise to in the foreseeable future?

Drawing on salient examples from mainstream education and the adult education literature, Dr Hyland clarifies the nature and extent of problems in store for us and provides an alternative conceptualisation and way forward for thinking about these issues. The relationship between professed educational philosophies and the wish to provide a high standard of service to the public is the underlying theme of this chapter, and it is suggested that this could usefully inform future policy direction at all levels of employee preparation and development in health care.

Introduction

Earl Russell (1994, p. 11) commented recently that:

> 'never since Oliver Cromwell dissolved the Rump Parliament in 1653 have we had a government which enjoyed worse relations with the professions than the government we have now.'

This state of affairs is a reflection and consequence of the widespread 'de-professionalisation' (Chitty & Simon 1993; Barton *et al.* 1994) that has occurred over the last decade or so in education and public service sectors as a result of central government's commitment to the ideologies of market forces and input/output efficiency and accountability. As Stronach (1995) has observed:

> 'professional life in Britain has developed a new vocabulary – innovation fatigue, early retirement, stress, overload and breaking point.'

Given all the recent 'policy hysteria' in areas such as health care, social work and education, it is little wonder that large numbers of professionals now feel 'over-stretched and under-valued'(Stronach 1995, p. 9).

There are a number of ways in which professional studies and practice have been affected by recent policy developments. Firstly, the culture of public service professions in fields such as health and education has been transformed through the gradual evolution, from the 1970s onwards, of a 'corporate state' characterised by order, nationalism and efficiency through which:

> 'production replaces consumption as the important preoccupation ... while efficiency becomes the overriding priority above the previous social democratic goals of equality and social justice.'
>
> (Ranson 1994, p. 43)

As Rustin (1994, pp. 76–7) has argued in relation to this tranformation of the public service ethic:

> 'To manage a budget and to achieve the public service equivalent of profit, has become the central concern of a whole stratum who previously thought of themselves as committed mainly to providing a social service. Seducing and cajoling the public sector middle class into the embrace of the market has been a key objective of public service reforms, potentially dissolving social democracy's core constituencies among professional workers as the attack on trade unions and public housing has sought to dissolve its larger mass base.'

Secondly, stemming from these radical shifts within the public sector, professional studies and education in general has been forced to change in order to accommodate the development of what Elliott (1993) has called the 'social market' model of education and training, according to which the:

> 'outcomes of professional learning are construed as quantifiable products which can be pre-specified in tangible and concrete form.'
>
> (Elliott 1993, pp. 16–17)

The chief vehicle for such change has been the competence-based education and training (CBET) strategy popularised in Britain through the work of the National Council for Vocational Qualifications (NCVQ). Although originally introduced as a way of accrediting work-based vocational skills, CBET has extended its remit throughout the system and now influences developments in professional studies and higher education (Hyland 1994). In the newly established Department for Education and Employment (DFEE), in which the industrial trainers seem to have extended their influence (Targett 1995), these utilitarian occupational trends may take on an even greater significance in the future.

The NCVQ model of CBET is highly suitable for effecting the de-professionalising and market forces changes referred to above. Its basic principle is that of:

> 'behaviourism with its implication that the significance of theoretical knowledge in training is a purely technical or instrumental one.'
>
> (Elliott 1993, p. 17)

The CBET model offers a 'production technology for commodifying professional learning for consumption' and also serves as an

> 'ideological device for eliminating value issues from the domains of professional practice and thereby subordinating them to political forms of control.'
>
> (Elliott 1993, pp. 23, 68)

Since, as I will be arguing, it is precisely the knowledge and ethical dimensions of professional theory and practice which are distinctive of and indispensable to the continuous renewal and rational development of professionalism in the teaching, health and other public service sectors, the impact of such de-professionalising forces needs to be resisted by educators and practitioners working in these domains. I intend to offer a critique of the NCVQ model of CBET before going on to suggest alternative strategies under the broad umbrella of what Elliott refers to as the 'practical science' (Elliott 1993, p. 17) model of professional development, which draws on action research and Schön's reflective practitioner tradition.

Although many of my references to practice are drawn from teacher education – particularly from my own experience in post-school and adult teacher education – I will also be at pains to demonstrate how the central issues and developments can be related to public sector professionalism in general. Both diagnosis and prescription are, therefore, intended to further a conception of 'extended professionalism' which is:

'rooted in a certain ethically conditioned appreciation and sensitivity to the needs of ... clients together with the informed wisdom and integrity to respond adequately to those needs.'

(Carr 1994, p. 47)

The limitations of competence-based education

It is generally accepted that the NCVQ approach has its origins in the performance-based teacher education movement which flourished in America in the 1960s (Tuxworth 1989), though this movement can itself be traced back to the 'social efficiency' theorists who were influential in the United States in the early 1900s. Theorists such as Snedden and Prosser criticised the educational practices of the time and recommended instead a system of 'utilitarian training which looks to individual efficiency in the world of work' (Wirth 1991, p. 57) as the overriding objective. John Dewey was to build his early reputation in criticising such narrowly utilitarian approaches just as, with the pendulum swings and recyclings of educational theory, contemporary liberal educators have similarly attacked the 'economic utility model' (Bailey 1984) which informs much of current vocational education and training (VET) policy and practice.

The NCVQ approach is based on the 'behaviourist' versions of CBET (Marshall 1991; Norris 1991) which involve the reduction of occupational roles to *statements of competence derived from a functional analysis of work roles*. This process involves 'breaking down the work role for a particular area into purposes and functions' (Mitchell 1989, p. 58) and the assessment of competence by means of 'performance criteria' which are

'determined or endorsed by a lead body with responsibility for determining, maintaining and improving national standards of performance in the sectors of employment where the competence is practised.'

(NCVQ 1991, p. 1)

The limitations and weaknesses of behaviourism as a learning theory have been well documented (Fontana 1984; Gross 1987) and I will not rehearse all of them here. In general terms, there is a tendency for behaviourist strategies to gloss over differences in learning styles, to stifle creative and intuitive learning and, through the reduction of learning objectives to prespecified measurable outcomes, to encourage a mechanical 'teaching to the test' approach which 'undervalues the importance of the learning process' (Tennant 1988, p. 120). Bull (1985) has questioned the 'moral validity' (p. 79) of using such strategies in educational contexts, and Marshall (1991) has argued that the 'functionalist and behavioural background' of the NCVQ approach has 'guaranteed that the model eventually produced is one-dimensional and prescriptive'. He concludes his critique with the assertion that:

> 'even the most radical behavioural psychologist would not now subscribe to the traditional view of learning so evident in the work of the NCVQ.'
>
> (Marshall 1991, pp. 61, 62)

An attachment to a discredited and psychologically dubious learning theory is by no means the only shortcoming of the NCVQ model of CBET. There is considerable confusion about what competence actually is (Ashworth & Saxton 1990) which has resulted in a 'plethora of opinions about competence and its definition' (Haffenden & Brown 1989, p. 139). The epistemological foundation of NVQs is as shaky as its psychological base (Barnett 1994; Hyland 1994) and there is still some uncertainty about whether competence really is, as originally conceived, about 'what people can do rather than what they know' (UDACE 1989, p. 6).

The recent changes in assessment and 'recontextualising' (Wolf 1990, p. 35) of competence – and the introduction of the General NVQs (Hyland 1993) – can be interpreted as an attempt to answer charges that the NCVQ approach is 'too occupationally specific' and 'minimalist' (Raggatt 1991, 1994). Trades union attitudes to the NCVQ system are, to say the least, lukewarm and ambivalent (Field 1991) and employers, who are supposed to be the leading players in this field, are either ignorant about or indifferent to what NVQs are offering (Field 1995; FEFC 1994). Callender's (1992) research on NVQs in the construction industry served to highlight some of these key shortcomings. Alongside the appalling ignorance, apathy and confusion of employers, she found NVQs which were:

> 'unduly limited in terms of the breadth of the activity they refer to and the demands they make on skills, knowledge and understanding. They are tending to squeeze out general job knowledge because of their emphasis on performance. This narrowness may therefore encourage rigidity rather than flexible application of skills. Consequently, some training providers feel that standards are falling'.
>
> (Callender 1992, p. 21)

All this must raise serious doubts about the appropriateness of CBET for occupational and professional development beyond the level of basic routine tasks (interestingly, over 90 per cent of the 350 000 NVQ certificates awarded up to the end of 1993 were at the lower levels of 1 and 2, (NCVQ 1994) equivalent to GCSE or below!).

The system is clearly not even delivering the goods in the area of work-based VET for which it was designed and, consequently, it appears rather foolhardy, if not bizarre, to try to apply CBET to contexts well outside this remit. As Marshall rightly points out, it would be 'ludicrous' to apply a model designed essentially for training basic skills 'to all levels of training' (Marshall 1991, p. 63). It would indeed be ludicrous, not to say disastrous to apply such a model to professional studies and professional development programmes and it is important to explain why this is so.

Learning and professional practice: beyond competence

In addition to all the flaws and shortcomings referred to, there is something decidedly odd about using the NCVQ system as a means of enhancing professional studies, upgrading VET or bringing about the 'learning society' when its chief proponents are insistent that 'NVQs have nothing whatsoever to do with training or learning programmes' (Fletcher 1991, p. 26). Similarly, we are informed that NVQs are 'independent of any specific course, programme or mode of learning' (NCVQ 1988, p. v) and 'firmly rooted in the functions of employment . . . without imposing an educational model of how people learn and behave' (Jessup 1991, p. 39).

However, no matter what the NCVQ rhetoric may *claim* about the independence of competence outcomes from learning programmes, the actual *implementation* of the system across a wide range of occupational sectors has resulted in a reduced curriculum, a loss of significant theoretical content, a restriction of student–teacher interaction and a de-skilling of work roles (Smithers 1993; Hyland 1994). All the evidence indicates that it is simply not viable to separate means and ends, learning and assessment in such an arbitrary manner. Moreover, how can a behaviourist-inspired CBET system, which is concerned only with *products* possibly service the needs of professional studies characterised by an emphasis on *processes*, growth and development?

Programmes of professional development in further education (Kerry & Tollitt-Evans 1992), higher education (Barnett 1994), social work (Winter 1992) and the caring professions generally (Hodkinson & Issitt 1995), though employing a diverse range of conceptual schemes and methodologies, tend to display a common distaste for technicist and behavioural models, preferring instead to found practice on ideas developed in the cognitive/humanistic tradition. Experiential learning theory is the broad term used to describe a range of activities which have been applied successfully to connect theory and practice in professional domains. It is unreservedly eclectic – drawing on the ideas of Dewey and Piaget as well as the critical theory of Habermas and Freire – though in its application to vocational and continuing professional education certain common characteristics have emerged.

Kolb (1993) offers a useful summary of the key features of experientialism, noting distinctive emphases on learning as a continuous activity grounded in experience, on the idea of an holistic process of adaptation through the resolution of conflicts, and on the conception of learning as a means of creating new knowledge rather than simply reinforcing and reifying existing epistemological traditions. Kolb aggregates all these ideas in his broad definition of experiential learning as 'the process whereby knowledge is created by the transformation of experience' (Kolb 1993, p. 155).

This conception of learning is fully in line with the prescriptions for active, critical and reflective learning found in all the mainstream accounts of professional studies. For those who support such a conception, behaviourist CBET must be anathema since it appears diametrically opposed to the fundamental tenets of the experiential tradition. Instead of an holistic framework, CBET fragments and atomises learning into measurable chunks; rather than valuing experience and process, CBET is concerned only with performance outcomes and, most significantly, instead of encouraging critical reflection on alternative perspectives related to changing situations, CBET offers a mono-cultural perspective based on the satisfaction of narrow performance criteria directed towards fixed and predetermined ends. Kolb covers all these shortcomings comprehensively in his observation that:

> 'When viewed from the perspective of experiential learning, the tendency to define learning in terms of outcomes can become a definition of non-learning, in the process sense that the failure to modify ideas and habits as a result of experience is maladaptive.'
>
> (Kolb 1993, p. 144)

It is difficult to see how such maladaptive systems of 'non-learning' can have any real value for professional studies which celebrate the continuous adaptation of ideas in response to learning gained from situational experience.

Moreover, in addition to the evident failure of CBET models to capture the sort of strategic, organisational and management skills typical of professional theory and practice, there is the danger that, in reducing professional knowledge and skill to simplistic competences, professional development may actually be *stifled* through the implication that competence is a once and for all achievement. It was just such a danger which prompted Eraut (1989), in examining the suitability of the NCVQ system for initial teacher education, to express the concern that, once trained, people might 'consider their competence as sufficient and ignore the need for further improvement' (p. 181). Such a failing takes on even more significance in the light of the empirical studies which indicate that, notwithstanding NCVQ public relations rhetoric, there is little or no evidence of progression on NVQ programmes (McHugh *et al.* 1993; Field 1995; Hyland 1994).

Mainstream CBET practices are, in fact, structurally incapable of furthering professional development beyond the level of collecting evidence to satisfy performance criteria. The problem is (and this is a supremely troublesome one for professional learning!) that CBET systems really only value the achievement or the *accreditation* of competence, not its *growth* over time. As Chown and Last (1993) note in their critique of the applications of CBET systems to post-school teacher education:

'the NCVQ model cannot acknowledge the growth of competence. It does not admit a change in competence which is not allied to a change in organisational function. There is, it would seem, no place for formally recognising the continuing development of teachers as competent practitioners unless they change roles – moving into management, mentorship or staff development.'

(Chown & Last 1993, pp. 21–2)

Another potentially problematic aspect of a CBET model based solely on employer-defined outcomes is the enormous power it gives managers to control and circumscribe the roles of workers. Of course, this is not necessarily sinister or totally undesirable though, unless we assume a kind of utopian state of benevolent employers, it may easily lead to one-sided and undemocratic power relations which are in no one's interests, especially not professionals and their clients.

Field (1991) has this in mind when he observes that the 'routinisation' and 'mechanistic behaviourism' of the NCVQ approach is ideally suited to the 'reinforcement of the divisions between different aspects of the work process', thus offering employers the means to 'narrow the scope of initiative and field of responsibility of each individual in her work' (Field 1991, pp. 49–50). In a similar vein, Edwards (1993) has argued that the rhetoric about open and flexible learning in work-based VET can be seen as 'another aspect of post-Fordism, strategically arranged to normalise a view of the future of work' by which 'persons will be disciplined into certain forms of behaviour and more readily managed within a social formation of structural inequality' (Edwards 1993, pp. 180, 185).

In addition, the key epistemological and ethical dimensions of practice – stressed in all the philosophical, sociological and psychological accounts of professionalism (Langford 1978; Larson 1977; Eraut 1994) – are seriously undervalued if not overlooked completely in the behaviourist CBET models. As mentioned already, knowledge is allowed to enter the picture in such systems only in so far that it promotes the collection of evidence to satisfy performance criteria. Knowledge belongs to 'the realm of inputs rather than outputs' and 'its introduction can only be justified if it is a necessary condition for generating the desired behavioural outcomes of learning' (Elliott 1993, p. 17). This is forcefully expressed by Mansfield (1990) in the assertion that we begin to 'recognise and locate knowledge in its rightful place' when we come to regard it 'as a source of evidence, together, with performance evidence' (Mansfield 1990, p. 21).

Although knowledge as evidence has some role to play in professional learning (in accrediting prior learning, certification, and so on), evidence gathering is not at the heart of professional theory and practice. Professional knowledge – as knowledge-in-use and situational understanding – is central to the 'practical science' models discussed below which stress the value of fostering reflective practice and the continuing drive for enhanced expertise. And this is not simply a question of legitimising professional work through the maintenance of a strong knowledge base, but the insistence that practical knowledge, research and reflection are indispensable to the work of professionals in education, health and the caring professions (Hodkinson & Issitt 1995).

Similarly, the inter- and intra-relationships between professionals and clients, and between professionals and colleagues, demand a high level of ethical and moral understanding which is simply ignored in behaviourist CBET systems which either serve to neutralise practice or reduce values to mechanistic competences. The obsession with collecting evidence to satisfy competence criteria is individualistic and is not able to accommodate the importance of teamwork and collegial collaboration in professional work (Ashworth 1992; Chown & Last 1993). Moreover, such technicist approaches to education and training do not acknowledge the extent to which professional skills and values are a product of joint social action developed through engagement in a complex set of interwoven social transactions (Wertsch 1991). As will be suggested in the later examination of the 'practical science' models, there is much to recommend the notion that the specifically *moral* aspects of professionalism are really what is distinctive of much practice and also what makes continuous professional development and enrichment possible.

Developments in professional studies

The 'de-professionalising' impact of CBET on educational studies in general, and teacher education in particular was mentioned in the introduction. Utilising Hoyle's (1983) analysis of professionalisation in terms of the distinction between *professionalism*, concerned with the 'improvement of status' and *professionality* (or professional development) connected with the 'improvement of skills' (Hoyle 1983, p. 45), it seems legitimate to argue that, until recently, these internal and external factors have been reasonably well balanced and complementary in the spheres of nursing, teaching and social work. Both the knowledge and skills base of such professions have been developed along with their enhanced status in the public domain.

However, in the wake of the trends mentioned earlier, coupled with the widespread vocationalisation of curricula and centralisation of control over the education system (Whitty 1990; Hyland 1991), there has been a narrowing of academic focus at all levels of the teaching profession, a de-skilling of the teaching role, and a corresponding loss of autonomy, status and morale (Tomlinson 1993; Barton *et al.* 1994).

Management competencies

Management competencies – particularly the widely-used management charter initiative model (Ramsay 1993) – have introduced technicist and behaviourist approaches into professional studies programmes in teaching, health and medical education (Challis *et al.* 1993). Such developments have, however, met with a high degree of resistance in certain spheres. Interestingly enough, professions within the health service – in spite of the last five traumatic years of NHS reforms in line with the social market model (Culyer 1995) – have managed to resist some of the worst features of the competence onslaught on professional studies. As in the sphere of initial school teacher education (Furlong 1995), although 'competences' are now part of the academic discourse within nursing and allied professions, the interpretation of competence is far more broadly-based and inclusive of professional values (Palmer *et al.* 1994) than, for example the Training and Development Lead Body (TDLB) standards which are being applied in further and adult education (Chown & Last 1993).

Certainly, in the light of the traditional role of higher education in validating certain professions (Eraut 1994), the move from a training base to an education base in the nursing profession through Project 2000 (UKCC 1986), seems to be both professionally supportive and prudent (even if it is also bizarrely contraindicative in the light of recent trends!) given the moves in the opposite direction within teaching and other spheres over the last decade or so.

However, there can be no doubt that the CBET 'outcomes' approach and the activities of the professional training lobby pose a threat to all types of professional learning and, though such programmes might, as Collins (1991) notes, serve the interests of management, they tend to marginalise vocational and professional skill and commitment. Professional teachers of all kinds are thus urged by Collins to mount a 'vigorous resistance to this destructive approach to education and training' (Collins 1991, p. 45). Edwards (1993) has suggested that educators who wish to counter the competence challenge must, in order to avoid being labelled as regressive Luddites, develop creative responses which incorporate detailed accounts of alternative conceptions of practice which are supported by relevant evidence and argument. The best way to do this is to examine the nature of professional learning and the theoretical underpinnings of practice.

Professional learning and practical science

Elliott (1993) has described three influential models of professional development and, although these are used principally to characterise mainstream trends in teacher education, they provide a useful framework for examining the nature of professional studies in general. In addition to the social market model associated with CBET already mentioned, there is a traditional 'platonic/rationalist' (Elliott 1993, p. 16) model which is embedded in higher education and stresses academic study and theoretical understanding as a way of developing rationally-autonomous professionals. It was the inadequacy of this model which, particularly in the field of initial teacher education, resulted in the development of the more practitioner-based, action research models developed from the 1970s onwards (Bridges 1995). Moreover, it has to be said that it has been the opacity of the traditional model and its lack of attention to public criteria and accountability which has allowed the competence challenge (Hodkinson & Issitt 1995) to damage professional studies so much in recent times. This is all the more unfortunate in that the top-down imposition of NCVQ aproaches has obscured the valuable developments that were taking place in practitioner and work-based professional studies which Elliott seeks to encapsulate in the 'practical science' model (Elliott 1993, p. 17).

Linked with action research and the teacher development tradition pioneered by Stenhouse in the 1970s (Stenhouse 1975), the 'practical science' model is incredibly eclectic, drawing on critical theory (Carr & Kemmis 1986), experiential learning (Kolb 1993), the research on vocational expertise (Chi *et al.* 1988) and the reflective practitioner model based on Schön's work (Schön 1987). The central ideas, which make use of the 'knowledge-in-use' and 'theories-in-action' devised initially by Argyris & Schön (1974) for developing and enhancing professional effectiveness, include such conceptions as:

- 'professional knowledge consists of reportoires of experienced cases which are stored in a practitioner's long-term memory and represent his or her stock of situational understandings'
- 'professional judgments and decisions are ethical and not just technical in character'
- 'systematic reflection by practitioners in their practical situations plays a central role in improving professional judgments and decisions.'

(Elliott 1993, pp. 67–8)

The importance of situational understanding was originally noted and emphasised in the work of Dreyfus (1981) in empirical studies of practical decision-making in the sphere of business management. Applied to professional studies in nurse education by Benner (1982), to the training of police officers by Elliott (1989) and to teacher education (Eraut 1994), this model consists of a five stage description of skill acquisition: novice, advanced beginner, competent, proficient and expert. It is interesting to note that, on this account, a 'competent' practitioner would only be around half way to the realisation of full potential in any particular occupational or professional sphere.

The significant feature of this approach to professional studies is the underlying assumption that learning needs to be seen as a continuous and ongoing process rather than a once and for all achievement. Just as the philosopher of education, R.S. Peters, suggested that to become educated was not to arrive at a destination but, rather, to travel with a different view (Peters 1966) so we can conceive of professional learning as a career-long process directed towards the continuous refinement and enrichment of knowledge, skills and expertise.

The concept of expertise – defined by Tennant (1991) as the 'knowledge and skill gained through sustained practice and experience' (p. 50) – has figured prominently in the professional studies field in recent years and there is now a substantial body of empirical work surrounding its applications. Summarising a range of such studies, Chi *et al.* (1988) identified a number of common characteristics, the key ones being that experts tended to excel in their own domains, had access to a body of systematically organised specialist knowledge, spent a lot of time analysing problems qualitatively and displayed strong self-monitoring skills. All these qualities match well with the reflective practitioner and practical science models of professionalism.

However, being an 'expert' is not simply a matter of attaining a higher level of technical efficiency than a novice or competent practitioner but requires the development of a perspective which includes an active concern with aims and consequences and full engagement in a process in which professionals continually monitor, evaluate and revise their own practice. The concepts of holistic action and 'professional artistry' (Jones 1995) serve to explain these aspects of the work of professionals and, as Eraut (1994) notes with teaching specifically in mind, that the 'actor image' is close to the reality of practice. He goes on to explain that:

> 'Technique is important for the actor but no performance can be analysed down to a set of distinct and separate skills. Interpretation and style are personal yet flexible, for the actor can play several different roles. Performance is improved by observation, discussion, reflection and experiment with only an occasional need for guided practice. Actors, however, have continuing opportunities to learn from each other...'
>
> (Eraut 1994, p. 37)

Professional expertise is not, however, just a matter of cognitive or intellectual development but relates to the affective (or emotional) dimensions of practice and the centrality of ethics and professional values. The nature of inter-relationships, between professionals and clients and the ethical bases and contexts of various practices, serve to place moral issues at the heart of professionalism in health, education and the caring services generally. In the context of nursing, Carper (1978) suggests that the 'ethical pattern of knowing' requires 'an understanding of different philosophical positions regarding what is good, what ought to be desired, what is right' (p. 21).

Similarly, in the sphere of teaching, Carr (1994) suggests that problems and situations call for a 'moral rather than a technical response' and seeks to characterise professional practice in terms of 'virtues rather than skills' (pp. 47, 48). He explains that:

> 'To speak of a bad plumber, for example, is by and large to identify someone who does a technically poor repair job rather than (say) overcharges, whereas talk of an unsatisfactory lawyer or general

practitioner is for the most part of someone who does not take proper time to understand his or her clients' needs in a proper spirit of care and concern ... Where concerns are professional, then, the emphasis is upon the ethically principled or moral quality of the response to the clients' needs...'

(Carr 1994, p. 47)

Sites of workplace learning and professional strategies

The developments in professional studies informed by the reflective practitioner model have resulted in a revival and reaffirmation of the importance of the *workplace* as the principal site of vocational and professional learning and development. However, the various strategies on offer – whether they relate to the 'coaching' schemes in industry (Slipais 1993), the 'preceptor' schemes in the health field (Kitchin 1993; Morton-Cooper & Palmer 1993) or the 'mentor' schemes in teacher education (Turner 1995) – though they may all be inspired by some form of commitment to experiential and work-based learning, differ in terms of organisation, culture and philosophical orientation. Moreover, these differences are of the first importance for they relate to the fundamental ethical bases of professional practice stressed earlier.

Differences between professional developments in the health service and in teacher education have already been noted though there are some interesting and significant parallels between intial training practices in the two domains (Booth *et al.* 1995). It is true that there is an overlap of both professional values and strategy in that the Project 2000 conception of locating learning within higher education involves the occupation of a position which, largely as a result of the imposition of centralised state policy, teacher education is being forced to vacate. However, this post-modernist fragmentation and fluidity (Sayers 1995) is not entirely negative in that it creates space for creative engagement with contemporary trends and ideological currents of change. Examples of such creative responses have been cited in connection with the strategies adopted to counter the competence challenge in education and social work (Winter 1992; Hodkinson & Issitt 1995). What is happening in mentorship and school-based teacher education schemes provides a vivid illustration of the nature of the struggle and contains some valuable lessons for professional studies in general.

There have been two main responses to the government policy of ensuring that initial teacher education is located predominantly within schools. The 'corporate' model (Bridges 1995, p. 69) based on the training schemes of large organisations, such as ICI and Sony, interprets the logic of the social market literally and makes the individual school the central unit of the delivery of education and training. This would be particularly popular in the case of opted-out, grant-maintained schools which have lost all links with the local education authority and have to purchase all services, including training and staff development, from external agencies. The weaknesses of this model have become evident in recent years (and were identified in a recent report by Ofsted inspectors, Tysome 1995): concentration on one institution tends to breed a parochialism of interests, a narrow institution-specific conception of theory and practice, and a loss of connection with the broader concerns and values of the profession. In terms of experiential learning, such a model can easily lead to an exclusively 'pragmatic' (Bridges 1995, p. 76), technicist and morally impoverished conception of professional practice.

Recognising these dangers, a number of schools and teacher education organisations have developed a more 'collaborative' model (Bridges 1995, pp. 70–72) which stresses the importance of maintaining the relationship between higher education institutions and clusters of schools. In this way, it is possible to offer trainees a much wider range of experience across schools and also to reinforce the central importance of the theoretical underpinnings of practice and the need to maintain a critical stance in relation to changes and developments in the field.

The critical evaluation of practice is, perhaps, more important than it has ever been in the present climate dominated by the 'impoverished policy process' described by Gipps (1993). The standard policy-making model is now one in which:

> 'think tanks promote policy through strong value assertions and then proceed directly to detailed descriptions. Argumentation is intuitive; there is an appeal at most to anecdotal evidence but not to research.'
>
> (Gipps 1993, p. 36)

Given this state of affairs the need for independent and critical thinking on the part of public service professionals takes on increasing importance. Professionals who become isolated within institutions are unlikely to be able to develop such capacities. Teachers working in opted-out schools, nurses working in NHS Trust hospitals and, since April 1993, further education lecturers employed in new corporate colleges (NATFHE 1992; Hyland & Turner 1995) are isolated from collegial values and influences and vulnerable to the managerialist policies of individual, and increasingly insular, institutions. Alienated in this way, there is less likelihood that critical discourse and alternative perpectives will come to inform the policy-making of an increasingly centralised bureaucracy dominated by technicist and instrumentalist ideological commitments.

Similarly, the 'individualistic' values associated with the social market approach to public service provision will flourish best if the strongly supportive NCVQ model is combined with workplace experiences – reinforced by league tables and competition between institutions – which celebrate corporate self-interest and eschew teamwork, collaboration and community service. This would be disastrous both for professionals and their clients since it would marginalise and perhaps even obscure the essential conception of professional practice as a *social* activity concerned with issues which require 'collective, rather than merely individual, action, (Barton *et al.* 1994, p. 540).

It is in this area that the ethical dimensions of professional practice need to be constantly renewed and reinforced. In spite of the individualism of the social market model of provision, the emergence of the 'learning organisation' has served to emphasise the importance of teamwork and collaboration at all levels in industry and the public services (Caldwell & Carter 1993). All this has resulted in the 'drive for a stronger culture of service in the public and private sector' (Caldwell & Carter 1993, p. 208) and the emergence of the mentorship and preceptorship schemes as paradigm models of development. However, though professionals may legitimately wish to endorse the 'pragmatic' reasons for supporting the new learning culture, in terms of promoting increased efficiency and improved client services, the ethical aspects of the service culture can also provide a cogent 'philosophical' argument against the more technicist, utilitarian and de-professionalising elements of recent trends in the public sector.

References

Argyris, C. & Schön, D. (1974) *Theory in Practice: Increasing Professional Effectiveness*. Jossey-Bass, San Francisco, CA.

Ashworth, P. (1992) Being competent and having 'competencies'. *Journal of Further and Higher Education*, **16**(3), 8–17.

Ashworth, P. & Saxton, J. (1990) On competence. *Journal of Further and Higher Education*, **14**(2), 3–15.

Bailey, C. (1984) *Beyond the Present and the Particular*. Routledge & Kegan Paul, London.

Barnett, R. (1994) *The Limits of Competence*. Open University Press, Buckingham.

Barton, L., Barrett, E., Whitty, G., *et al.* (1994) Teacher education and professionalism in England: some merging issues. *British Journal of Sociology of Education*, **15**(4), 529–43.

Benner, P. (1982) From novice to expert. *American Journal of Nursing*, **82**(3), 402–407.

Black, H. & Wolf, A. (eds) (1990) *Knowledge and Competence: Current Issues in Training and Education.* Careers and Occupational Information Centre, Sheffield.

Booth, M., Bradley, H., Hargreaves, D.H., *et al.* (1995) Training of doctors in hospitals: a comparison with teacher education. *Journal of Education for Teaching,* **21**(2), 145–62.

Bridges, D. (1995) School-based teacher education. In: *Issues in Mentoring,* (eds T. Kerry & A. Shelton Mayes). Routledge/Open University, London.

Bull, H. (1985) The use of behavioural objectives. *Journal of Further and Higher Education,* **9**(1), 74–80.

Burke, J.W. (ed.) (1989) *Competency Based Education and Training.* Falmer Press, Lewes.

Caldwell, B.J. & Carter, E.M.A. (eds) (1993) *The Return of the Mentor: Strategies for Workplace Learning.* Falmer Press, London.

Callender, C. (1992) *Will NVQs Work? Evidence from the Construction Industry.* Institute of Manpower Studies, University of Sussex.

Carper, B.A. (1978) Fundamental patterns of knowing in nursing. *Advances in Nursing Science,* **1**(1), 13–23.

Carr, D. (1994) Educational enquiry and professional knowledge: towards a Copernican revolution. *Educational Studies,* **20**(1), 33–52.

Carr, W. & Kemmis, S. (1986) *Becoming Critical: Education, Knowledge and Action Research.* Falmer Press, Lewes.

Challis, H., Underwood, T. & Joesbury, H. (1993) Assessing specified competences in medical undergraduate training. *Competence and Assessment,* Issue 22, 6–9.

Chi, M., Glaser, R. & Farr, M. (1988) *The Nature of Expertise.* Lawrence Erlbaum Associates, Hillsdale, NJ.

Chitty, C. & Simon, B. (eds) (1993) *Education Answers Back.* Lawrence & Wishart, London.

Chown, A. & Last, J. (1993) Can the NCVQ model be used for teacher training? *Journal of Further and Higher Education,* **17**(2), 15–26.

Collins, M. (1991) *Adult Education as Vocation.* Routledge, London.

Culyer, T. (1995) Cure at a cost; medicine synthesis. *Times Higher Education Supplement,* 20.1.95.

Dreyfus, S.E. (1981) *Formal Models v. Human Situational Understanding: Inherent Limitations on the Modelling of Business Expertise.* US Air Force Office of Scientific Research, University of California, Berkeley.

Edwards, R. (1993) The inevitable future? Post-Fordism in work and learning. In: *Adult Learners, Education and Training,* (eds R. Edwards, A. Sieminski & D. Zeldin). Routledge/Open University, London.

Elliott, J. (1989) Appraisal of performance or appraisal of persons. In: *Rethinking Appraisal and Assessment,* (eds H. Simon & J. Elliott). Open University, Milton Keynes.

Elliott, J. (ed.) (1993) *Reconstructing Teacher Education.* Falmer Press, London.

Eraut, M. (1989) Initial teacher training and the NCVQ model. In: *Competency Based Education and Training,* (ed. J.W. Burke). Falmer Press, Lewes.

Eraut, M. (1994) *Developing Professional Knowledge and Competence*. Falmer Press, London.

FEFC (1994) *National Vocational Qualifications in the FE Sector in England*. Further Education Funding Council, Coventry.

Field, J. (1991) Competency and the predagogy of labour. *Studies in the Education of Adults*, **23**(1), 41–52.

Field, J. (1995) Reality testing in the workplace: are NVQs 'employment-led'?. In: *The Challenge of Competence; Professionalism through Vocational Education and Training*, (eds P. Hodkinson & M. Issitt). Cassell, London.

Fletcher, S. (1991) *NVQs, Standards and Competence*. Kogan Page, London.

Fontana, D. (ed.) (1984) *Behaviourism and Learning Theory in Education*. Scottish Academic Press, Edinburgh.

Furlong, J. (1995) The limits of competence: a cautionary note on circular 9/92. In: *Issues in Mentoring*, (eds T. Kerry & A. Shelton Mayes). Routledge/Open University, London.

Gipps, C. (1993) Policy-making and the use and misuse of evidence. In: *Education Answers Back*, (eds C. Chitty & B. Simon). Lawrence & Wishart, London.

Gross, R.D. (1987) *Psychology*. Edward Arnold, London.

Haffenden, I. & Brown, A. (1989) Towards the implementation of NVQs in further education colleges. In: *Competency Based Education and Training*, (ed. J.W. Burke). Falmer Press, Lewes.

Hodkinson, P. & Issitt, M. (eds) (1995) *The Challenge of Competence; Professionalism through Vocational Education and Training*. Cassell, London.

Hoyle, E. (1983) The professionalization of teachers: a paradox. In: *Is Teaching A Profession?* (ed. P. Gordon). Institute of Education, London.

Hyland, T. (1991) Taking care of business: vocationalism, competence and the enterprise culture. *Educational Studies*, **17**(1), 77–87.

Hyland, T. (1993) GNVQs – putting learning back into VET. *Educa*, No. 134, 10–11.

Hyland, T. (1994) *Competence, Education and NVQs: Dissenting Perspectives*. Cassell, London.

Hyland, T. & Turner, M. (1995) Chasing Cinderella: principals' perspectives on FE incorporation. *Educational Change and Development*, **16**(2), 41–7.

Jessup, G. (1991) *Outcomes: NVQs the Emerging Model of Education and Training*. Falmer Press, London.

Jones, J. (1995) Professional artistry and child protection: towards a reflective, holistic practice. In: *The Challenge of Competence; Professionalism through Vocational Education and Training*, (eds P. Hodkinson & M. Issitt). Cassell, London.

Kerry, T. & Shelton Mayes, A. (eds) (1995) *Issues in Mentoring*. Routledge/Open University, London.

Kerry, T. & Tollitt-Evans, J. (1992) *Teaching in Further Education*. Blackwell Publishers, Oxford.

Kitchin, S. (1993) Preceptorship in hospitals. In: *The Return of the Mentor: Strategies for Workplace Learning*, (eds B.J. Caldwell & E.M.A. Carter). Falmer Press, London.

Kolb, D. (1993) The process of experiential learning. In: *Culture and Processes of Adult Learning*, (eds M. Thorpe, R. Edwards & A. Hanson). Routledge/Open University, London.

Langford, G. (1978) *Teaching as a Profession*. Manchester University Press, Manchester.

Larson, M.S. (1977) *The Rise of Professionalism: A Sociological Analysis*. University of California Press, Berkeley, CA.

McHugh, G., Fuller, A. & Lobley, D. (1993) *Why Take NVQs?* Centre for the Study of Training and Education, Lancaster University.

Mansfield, B. (1990) Knowledge, evidence and assessment. In: *Knowledge and Competence: Current Issues in Training and Education*, (eds H. Black & A. Wolf). Careers and Occupational Information Centre, Sheffield.

Marshall, K. (1991) NVQs: an assessment of the 'outcomes' approach in education and training. *Journal of Further and Higher Education*, **15**(3), 56–64.

Mitchell, L. (1989) The definition of standards and their assessment. In: *Competency Based Education and Training*, (ed. J.W. Burke). Falmer Press, Lewes.

Morton-Cooper, A. & Palmer, A. (1993) *Mentoring & Preceptorship: A Guide to Support Roles in Clinical Practice*. Blackwell Science, Oxford.

NATFHE (1992) *The Community College*. National Association of Teachers in Further and Higher Education, London.

NCVQ (1988) *Initial Criteria and Guidelines for Staff Development*. National Council for Vocational Qualifications, London.

NCVQ (1991) *Criteria for National Vocational Qualifications*. National Council for Vocational Qualifications, London.

NCVQ (1994) *NVQ Monitor – Winter 1993/94*. National Council for Vocational Qualifications, London.

Norris, N. (1991) The trouble with competence. *Cambridge Journal of Education*, **21**(3), 331–41.

Palmer, A., Burns, S. & Bulmer, C. (1994) *Reflective Practice in Nursing: The Growth of the Professional Practitioner*. Blackwell Science, Oxford.

Peters, R.S. (1966) *Ethics and Education*. Allen & Unwin, London.

Raggatt, P. (1991) Quality assurance and NVQs. In: *Change and Intervention: Vocational Education and Training*, (eds P. Raggatt & L. Unwin). Falmer Press, London.

Raggatt, P. (1994) Implementing NVQs in colleges; progress, perceptions and issues. *Journal of Further and Higher Education*, **18**(1), 59–74.

Ramsay, J. (1993) The hybrid course: competences and behaviourism in higher education. *Journal of Further and Higher Education*, **17**(3), 70–89.

Ranson, S. (1994) *Towards the Learning Society*. Cassell, London.

Russell, C. (1994) Professions in the firing line. *Times Higher Education Supplement*, 20.5.94.

Rustin, M. (1994) Unfinished business – from Thatcherite modernisation to incomplete modernity. In: *Altered States: Postmodernism, Politics, Culture*, (ed. M. Perryman). Lawrence & Wishart, London.

Sayers, S. (1995) The value of community. *Radical Philosophy*, **69**, 2–4.

Schön, D. (1987) *Educating the Reflective Practitioner: Towards a New Design for Teaching and Learning in the Professions.* Jossey-Bass, San Francisco, CA.

Slipais, S. (1993) Coaching in a competency-based training system: the experience of the Power Brewing Company. In: *The Return of the Mentor: Strategies for Workplace Learning,* (eds B.J. Caldwell & E.M.A. Carter). Falmer Press, London.

Smithers, A. (1993) *All Our Futures: Britain's Education Revolution.* Channel 4 Television 'Dispatches' Report on Education, London.

Stenhouse, L. (1975) *An Introduction to Curriculum Research and Development.* Open University Press, Milton Keynes.

Stronach, I. (1995) Policy hysteria. *Forum,* **37**(1), 9–10.

Targett, S. (1995) Shephard picks her men. *Times Higher Education Supplement,* 4.8.95.

Tennant, M. (1988) *Psychology and Adult Learning.* Routledge, London.

Tennant, M. (1991) Expertise as a dimension of adult development. *New Education,* **13**(1), 49–55.

Tomlinson, J. (1993) *The Control of Education.* Cassell, London.

Turner, M. (1995) The role of mentors and teacher tutors in school-based teacher education and induction. In: *Issues in Mentoring,* (eds T. Kerry & A. Shelton Mayes). Routledge/Open University, London.

Tuxworth, E. (1989) Competence based education and training: background and origins. In: *Competency Based Education and Training,* (ed. J.W. Burke). Falmer Press, Lewes.

Tysome, T. (1995) In-school training limited. *Times Higher Education Supplement,* 18.8.95.

UDACE (1989) *Understanding Competence.* Unit for the Development of Adult Continuing Education, Leicester.

UKCC (1986) *Project 2000: A New Preparation for Practice.* United Kingdom Central Council for Nursing, Midwifery and Health Visiting, London.

Wertsch, J. (1991) *Voices of the Mind.* Harvester Wheatsheaf, London.

Whitty, G. (1990) The new Right and the National Curriculum: state control or market forces? In: *New Curriculum – National Curriculum,* (ed. B. Moon). Hodder & Stoughton, London.

Winter, R. (1992) 'Quality management' or the 'educative workplace': alternative versions of competence-based education. *Journal of Further and Higher Education,* **16**(3), 100–15.

Wirth, A.G. (1991) Issues in the vocational-liberal studies controversy (1900–1917). In: *Education for Work* (ed. D. Corson). Multilingual Matters, Clevedon.

Wolf, A. (1990) Unwrapping knowledge and understanding from standards of competence. In: *Knowledge and Competence: Current Issues in Training and Education,* (eds H. Black & A. Wolf). Careers and Occupational Information Centre, Sheffield.

7

Funding Issues in Education and Training

Margaret Bamford

This chapter examines the costs and processes involved in managing education and training budgets, and will be a helpful source of information and guidance to those attempting to disentangle and interpret policy guidelines regarding current and proposed funding arrangements here in the UK, particularly with regard to the formation of formal partnerships between education and service providers. The logistics and local politics of communicating problems and strategies to those indirectly (but often influentially) involved in making decisions over training and educational provision are also addressed, possibly in the hope of crossing over the traditionally perceived education–practice divide *which currently pervades the literature in health care both nationally and internationally.*

Introduction

Professional education and training is fundamental to producing a quality health service. It is essential in supporting innovation and change, and there has probably not been another time in the life of the National Health Service (NHS) when innovation and change have been so rapid and so high on the agenda. It is also important to know that here in the UK, £756 million is spent by the NHS on non-medical education each year. A further £352 million is spent on postgraduate medical and dental education (PGMDE), (NHSE 1995). This is big business, and does not take into account other money spent on education and training by employers.

Education and training is an important feature of the NHS. Although there has always been a strong partnership with higher education, a large proportion of education and training has been undertaken on NHS premises. There is now a move towards large groups of employees, i.e. nurses, midwives, physiotherapists and others, being educated in the higher education sector. There will, however, still be a need to provide some accommodation and facilities in the foreseeable future in the workplace, in order to maintain the high level of skill and expertise necessary in organisations with the range of scope of activity currently expected of health care providers.

Organisations such as the NHS, which are in a constant state of growth and development, need to evolve into learning organisations (Senge 1990; Pearn 1995). Senge (1990, p. 14) describes a learning organisation as:

'. . . an organisation that is continually expanding its capacity to create its future. For such an organisation, it is not enough merely to survive. "Survival learning" or what is more often termed "adaptive learning" is important – indeed it is necessary. But for a learning organisation "adaptive learning" must be joined by "generative learning", learning that enhances our capacity to create.'

There is a need for establishments to have an ongoing commitment to education and training and for each employee to develop a philosophy of life-long learning (UKCC 1995). An organisation which needs to react to a changing direction or environment quickly, needs to be supported by a responsive and flexible workforce. The rapidity of change does mean that there is an onus on the employing organisation to support and nurture staff, not only to maintain their level of skill and competence, but also to underpin this with a sound knowledge base provided through appropriate educational and continuing educational experience (Perry 1995).

The sweeping changes outlined in EL(94)71, (NHSE 1994a), will affect employees other than medical staff. This has already been demonstrated during the adjustments being made to the hours that junior doctors can work. As junior doctors work less hours and are involved in more directed educational programmes, this means that there will be opportunities to review skill mix in clinical areas. This then places an additional education and training requirement on other members of staff, and on the organisation as a whole. The opportunities arising out of this requirement are tremendous, but there does need to be an infrastructure which can support these developments, and a strategy which will facilitate change in each employing NHS Trust.

The range and type of education and training in the NHS therefore varies from that which is profession specific, through management and finance, to general requirements for physical handling and moving and health and safety. This is a wide remit, and most of that provided on site in Trusts is, and will be, of a continuing and expanding nature.

In any organisation which demonstrates the complexity of the NHS, there will be a need to provide education and training. This will continually update and improve the stock of knowledge and skill necessary to provide a safe and progressive service to the community. In addition to the need to provide continuous professional education, there is a need to provide the necessary knowledge and skills which will facilitate the management of the NHS. The NHS is as complex and diverse a business as any in the UK, and already must spend a considerable amount on education and training to support the management and functioning of the organisation (Drucker 1990; Pearn 1995).

Historical funding of education and training

Funding of education and training is, of course, a major consideration both at central government level and locally. Costings are now being identified in partnership with the higher education sector by means of the tendering process for nurse and midwifery education together with education and training for professionals allied to medicine. These costs are not a true reflection of the total costs of education and training. They only reflect the institutional elements of education and training, rather than the full costs, which contain a considerable input by service providers. Some early work done by Goodwin and Bosanquet (1986) for the Royal College of Nursing identified the following costs (based on 1982/3 prices):

'(a) The estimated cost of training a RN under the School of Nursing System is about £8750 over their three-year training period (£21 050 net of replacement cost of £12 300).

(b) The estimated cost of training a RN via degree courses is about £17 350 over their four-year training period (£23 000 net of replacement cost of £6150).

(c) The estimated cost of training a RN in diploma courses is about £10 250 over their three-year training period (£14 350 net of replacement cost of £4100). If such RNs proceed onto one year degree conversion courses, their overall costs rise to about £13 800 (£19 950 net of replacement cost of £6150).'

(Goodwin & Bosanquet 1986, p. 1).

These costs were based on:

- *formal costs* – direct teaching costs and maintenance allowances
- *informal costs* – manpower costs incurred due to the teaching role of ward based staff
- *replacement costs* – the work that the student nurses do, and the cost of replacing them.

This is now old research in that the world has moved on, but if these were the costs of nurse education, what were the costs of the rest of the workforce? Also will they have changed significantly in proportional terms over the last ten years? The only surety is that the cost will have gone up! This is important for the future, the costs that are being looked at now for example do not include one of the elements included by Goodwin and Bosanquet. The missing element is the informal cost, the manpower cost incurred due to the teaching role of ward-based staff. This would be an interesting exercise to replicate, and perhaps from a service provision point of view extend to all learners in the clinical environment – nurses, doctors, professions allied to medicine, managers, health care assistants. What is the financial cost, has it been budgeted for and would it affect contract prices?

The National Audit Office (1992) gave some other figures, figures which related again only to nursing but which are, nevertheless, interesting, and could be extrapolated with imagination:

- In England, the NHS employs 400 000 nurses at a cost of £5 billion per year.
- Each year the NHS recruits 20 000 nurses to replace retirees and leavers.
- 50 000 student nurses are undergoing pre-registration education annually, at a cost of £600 million.

The National Audit Office felt that there could be a reduction in education and training costs particularly for Project 2000 students by local health service employers giving:

'greater priority to increasing the proportion of potential future vacancies filled by qualified nurse returners.'

(National Audit Office 1992, p. 3).

To some extent this must be happening, with the reduction in student commissions across England. In many instances it could be less qualified staff who will be filling the gaps rather than qualified returners, who may be too expensive to employ.

The cost of recruiting qualified nurse returners must also be taken into account. There will be the need to recruit the right sort of person, with the right sort of experience, and also have in place arrangements for the right sort of ongoing education and training (Jarrold 1994). The NHS is a fast changing organisation, and people who have taken a break of just a few years would find some areas of work considerably changed. This does not only apply to nurses, but to all professional staff. The difficulties of keeping abreast of professional developments cannot be over emphasised, and of course there is a financial cost element to be borne.

Why do we need to change?

Historically, funding for education and training of nurses and midwives was part of a locally held budget at the then district health authority (DHA). This budget was managed by the senior nurse manager at district level, in partnership with the director of nurse education. The whole purpose of the budget was to assist in meeting the education and workforce needs within the DHA. The focus was not specifically education and training, and of course the budget was 'soft'. This means that the budget could be manipulated, it could be moved and used in alternative ways, it was not prescribed and rigid as other budgets could be. A shortfall in finances in a DHA could result in an intake of students being cut. It became apparent that this was not a useful way to manage workforce planning for such a dynamic business as the NHS, particularly with the reforms that were being envisaged, and planned for the future. Decisions were very much at a local level, and did not take into account other local needs, i.e. community, private sector, let alone regional and national needs.

Working Paper 10 (WP 10)

The 1989 white paper *Working for Patients* (DoH 1989) launched a series of working papers, tenth in this series was a paper which addressed the issue of pre-registration education and training for health professionals. The paper excluded doctors and dentists. The focus was very definitely on pre-registration or recordable qualifications. This meant tht community psychiatric nurses and community mental handicap nurses could be included, as well as conversion and other second recordable courses (Anon 1991). At that time in many regions, school nurse and practice nurse education and training was excluded.

The principal aim of WP 10 was to bring about a level playing field within the newly emerging internal market. This was done with the intention that all parties would be treated the same. The money that a directly managed unit (DMU) or Trust had been putting into education and training (under the WP 10 criteria), would be returned to them in full for the first year of the exercise for purchasing their WP 10 needs. It was felt to be unrealistic to include primary training costs in contract prices, as this would put some people at a disadvantage in deciding on contract price. The current spending on pre-registration education and training was identified for each Trust and DMU, and that money was withheld in the annual allocation, but held at the regional health authority (RHA). This was then to be a pool of money to bid against to support WP 10 education and training requests. The intention was to secure a supply of trained health professionals to meet the needs of all health providers, both in the NHS and in the rapidly emerging independent sector.

It quickly became apparent to all parties in the WP 10 arrangement that there were no accurate or robust mechanisms for costing education and training. Workforce planning at that stage was unsophisticated and very local, and did not really take into account the new developing areas of care, and the wider national needs.

The whole process of contracting for education and training was new and people had to develop expertise and knowledge as they went along. This new approach was needed because of the issues which have been identified previously and because the work of the NHS was, and is, changing. From 1 April 1993, the responsibility for funding allocations of professional education and training also moved to the RHAs from the English National Board, (NHSE 1994c). At the same time funding for teachers of nursing and midwifery education programmes moved. This meant that all funding associated with nursing and midwifery education was centrally held at the RHA. It is interesting to think about this in relation to the historical arrangements for funding. Now the money is in one pot, how will it be managed? How will it be allocated? What will be the professional input into decision-making?

Contracting for education and training has gained in sophistication. Colleges of nursing and midwifery have moved into higher education, or are about to do so, and the RHAs have drawn up contracts with higher education to provide qualified health professionals over a five-year period. Imagine the arena in which all this has taken place; massive change in the NHS; massive change in higher education; colleges of nursing and midwifery merging into higher education, to become an integral part of those institutions. No wonder it has taken some time to get to where we are, which is at the beginning of a new process – education and training consortia.

Consortia for education and training

Consortia are groups of Trusts, health authorities, other health employers and interested parties who will come together for the purpose of identifying education and training needs for a locality. Consortia have been identified as the way to move forward within the WP 10 framework, and an outline of their role and responsibilities was given in Chapter 7 of *Managing the New NHS: Functions and Responsibilities in the New NHS* (NHSE 1994b). The broad outlines have been given some substance by Ken Jarrold in a subsequent publication (NHSE 1995).

Consortia are necessary because of the decision to abolish the RHAs, and create regional offices (ROs). These ROs will be part of the new NHS Executive (NHSE) and be directly linked to the centre rather than having the relationship and authority of the RHAs. The total budget will be many millions, and will need careful management to maximise its potential for the health of the nation.

Chapter 7 of *Managing the New NHS* (NHSE 1994b) entitled 'Human Resources', explains how workforce planning and commissioning of education training will work in the future. The NHSE will set a framework within which health authorities and Trusts will have an increasing role in identifying education and training. At RO level a regional education and development group (REDG) will be established which will include representatives of the regional consortia and the postgraduate dean.

Initially, and for the immediate future, ROs will hold the budget for non-medical education and training and will also be responsible for negotiating contracts around education and training. The consortia will produce purchasing plans for education and training for the consideration of the REDG. The REDG will be expected to liaise with the various professions and the education providers in confirming and setting the arrangements.

The budget to support this activity will be drawn from a national levy on health authorities. The level of the levy will be set by the NHSE and will initially reflect current spending on education and training. The responsibility for ensuring adequacy of supply will continue to rest with the NHSE, and initially they will contract directly for the smaller specialised staff groups. There may be opportunities in the future for movement in the levy in response to service needs, for example the educational requirement subsequent to major national initiatives such as day case surgery.

In the longer term it is expected that responsibility for budget-holding and negotiation of contracts will be devolved to the consortia. The RO, advised by the REDG, will be responsible for validating the consortia's purchasing plans, and will where it is necessary, arbitrate between parties. Consortia will be gradually brought into the purchasing mechanisms for medical and dental education. Initially they will provide advice and information on workforce requirements for doctors, and also on local purchasing of medical education and training. It is expected that there will be other areas of education and training funded from WP 10 in the future. Management, personal and organisational development will be part of that future arrangement.

Consortia will allow for the development of a feeling of trust and a common understanding of the direction and focus of education and training in a locality. The people involved will be working together to identify how best to spend the money in the budget for the benefit of the communities which they serve. There will be the opportunity to develop local ownership of new developments and initiatives which will very much focus on the needs of the population. Opportunities to move forward to a new agenda of education and training based on those local needs and developments, focusing on purchasing and business plans, will quickly become apparent.

A new dialogue will be developed to identify need, and within this there will be opportunities for negotiation, and a strengthening of communication. This opportunity will bring other key purchasers of education and training into the debate, and should allow for a greater understanding of the issues surrounding education and training in a much wider health arena, across sectarian divides. This should ultimately lead to improved care and continuity of care for patients and clients.

Local consortia must work; there is a desperate need for all players to get involved in planning for the future. Taking into account the range and breadth of work which is done in the NHS there is a need to have education and training programmes which will meet those needs; quickly, effectively and efficiently. For too long the NHS has muddled through on the provision of education and training, it has been left to the very local whims of DHAs. Now consideration must be given to business plans, health commissioning, and the public/private provision of health care. This is the first time there has been such a strong steer from the centre on this issue. Of course, a more cynical person could say that it is the development of a strong business base in order to move that base from the health sector to the education sector. It should not be forgotten however, that a large and important input into the education and training programmes is practical experience.

The timetable for developments was outlined in EL(95)27 (NHSE 1995). Between April 1995 and March 1996:

'• formal arrangements begin, "shadow working" continues;
• non-medical workforce planning "owned" by consortia but supported by ROs;
• during the transitional phase, consortia ratify workforce planning proposals worked up by ROs and passed to the REDG;
• ROs continue to hold the budget and contract for all stage groups;
• for PGMDE consortia start to provide advice to Postgraduate Deans on workforce planning and, for example, local educational arrangements for junior doctors.'

(NHSE 1995)

This is a huge agenda to implement in such a short space of time, particularly as both the Department of Health and the ROs are working through such huge re-organisational changes.

From April 1996 onward it is expected:

'• the levy system [be] introduced;
• for NMET [non-medical education and training], ROs begin to devolve budget-holding and contracting to consortia when the latter meet explicit criteria for taking on these responsibilities;
• ROs may retain responsibilities for commissioning education for certain small staff groups;
• REDGs (through negotiation and agreement) reconcile proposals from consortia to ensure they are coherent and consistent;
• Postgraduate Deans remain responsible for commissioning PGMDE, but continue to be advised by consortia and be members of REDGs.'

(NHSE 1995)

This arrangement allows for a hierarchical structure which will support the workforce and planning work. The work will be done at grassroots where it needs to be done, reviewed against a regional need and finally against a national agenda. Including medical and dental education this allows for more work to be done on skill mix issues.

Examples of consortia for education and training based on EL(95)27, (NHSE 1995)

Membership of a consortia executive group

Chief executives (CE) of provider units (or nominees)
Chief executives of commissioning authorities (or nominees)
Representatives of GPs
Representatives of GPFHs
Representatives of social services
Representatives of independent sector
Representatives of voluntary sector
Regional office representative
Nominee of the regional postgraduate dean (RPGD) (it would seem sensible to have the RPGD represented if the consortia are to give advice on medical needs)

The membership of the executive group is prescribed and there will be allowances for local needs to be met. This listing is slightly different to the list in the Executive Letter (NHSE 1995), in that it includes a slightly broader representation. It is possible that in most consortia there will be arrangements made for a wider grouping of interested people. The range of people with the exception of the representative of the RPGD are as described in the Executive Letter. It is anticipated that by involving this range of people in the decision-making process at local levels there will be greater involvement and commitment. There will also be a greater understanding of the professional education and training needs in a locality, and therefore greater strength in the workforce planning process.

The consortia executive group will have responsibility for providing strategic direction for meeting local education and training needs within the broad policy framework of the RO and the NHSE. They will be responsible for collecting and collating workforce plans of constituent members of the consortia, and providing information on the demand for newly-qualified staff for the future, initially for a five-year period. They will need to take into account the needs of non-hospital and social services partners when doing workforce planning. This group will eventually commission education directly from education providers, taking into account quality, admission policies, and 'fitness for purpose'. They will act in an advisory capacity to the REDG on the number and types of doctors needed in the consortia's locality, and ensure mechanisms are in place to support the educational contracting process within the consortia.

There will possibly be sub-groups of the executive group of the consortia, who will be more actively involved in areas of specialism, these could include:

- a professional advisory group (PAG)
- a workforce planning group (WPG)
- a finance group (FG).

A *professional advisory group* (PAG), which would have its membership drawn from professional nursing and midwifery leads of all the member Trusts, and health authorities and includes representatives from physiotherapy, occupational therapy, radiography, management and finance development groups. The aim of this group would be to support the activities of the consortia and contribute to professional education and training in the Trusts who are members of the consortia. They could be responsible for advising the consortia on issues related to education and training which affect the delivery of service, and also advising on changes in service which will impact on the delivery of education and training programmes.

The PAGs will be able to identify the range and extent of education provision that the Trusts require and are prepared to support, and be in a position to receive information on quantitative and qualitative data from educational providers relating to student activity. They would have a very strong lead in advising on the outcomes of education and training programmes in relation to 'fitness for purpose', and they will be able to liaise closely with RO colleagues on professional issues.

Another sub-group could be a *workforce planning group* (WPG). This group would be made up of human resource representatives from the member Trusts, together with a representative from the PAG, and financial advice. The contribution of this group would be to support the activities of the consortia, through their special understanding of workforce planning issues within the NHS. They could be responsible for advising the consortia on all issues related to workforce planning; and collecting and collating data from all Trust members, using a standard method. Their ability to inform purchasing intentions of the consortia for education and training will be an important area of work. Monitoring outcomes of education and training commissions, in order to inform future planning will be essential. They could liaise closely with PAG in relation to professional perspectives of outcomes of commissions, and also liaise with RO colleagues on workforce issues.

A final sub-group will be a *finance group* (FG) which would have representatives of all the Trusts with a special interest in financial issues. Their aim will be to support the activities of the consortia by their special knowledge and understanding of the NHS financial requirements. This group's responsibilities will be for providing financial statements for the executive group and monitoring spending within the consortia. They will receive commissioning intentions from the workforce planning group in order to provide supporting evidence for the executive group, and liaise with RO colleagues in financial issues.

How will it work/evolve?

Consortia will need to have a clear idea of how they will work and move forward. There will be a need to have a central concept of education and training which supports organisational development, and meets the requirements of the various business plans. Education and training developments will need to bridge traditional inter-sectoral boundaries for the benefit of patients and clients. This development should lead to the establishment of common standards across the consortia for clinical practice, management and education. There is the possibility of a reduction in duplication of provision of education and training, which would lead to a reduction in overhead costs, which could be achieved by sharing facilities and expertise. There will be increased opportunity for intra- and inter-disciplinary education and training which is a philosophy common to many professional groups (DoH 1993, 1994; Horder 1995; Funnell 1995; SCOPME 1995), also a potential of sharing of resources for education and training across disciplines, directorates and departments.

This development should lead to improved communication across the consortia on education and training issues. There should also be opportunities for an increase in collaborative research, through a much better educated workforce, which respects each member's contribution.

Comments and things to think about in developing consortia

In all instances it will be important to seek as wide as possible a representation of chief executives (CEs), professional, financial, human resource and contracting input to the executive group. CEs will need to bear this in mind if nominating someone to represent them on the executive group.

The contribution of the chairperson of this group requires very careful consideration, bearing in mind the amount of work that needs to be done to develop the executive groups into a productive unit by the start date of 1996. The problem is compounded by the fact that all Trusts at the moment probably have different mechanisms for workforce planning, and different development agendas, and very heavy work loads. There will be a need to establish a small team of people who will manage this process on behalf of the executive group. There will be a need for a manager, probably on a half-time basis, with experience of contracting; there will also be a need for secretarial support, again a half-time appointment perhaps. Financial support will be needed, as will human resource support, both of these could come from member Trusts. Funding for this small team would need to be sought from WP 10.

A common workforce planning tool would be needed across all the member Trusts. There may be a development cost associated with this, but this could perhaps be a pan-regional development with costs therefore potentially being reduced. Relationships with RO colleagues will need to be developed, bearing in mind the process of change that has been going on at the RHA/RO, and that this is a major piece of work being given to Trusts who have limited experience of this type of work. Whoever takes over the 'management' role of looking after the business as a whole will need to demonstrate a 'loyalty' to all Trusts and the establishment of sound communication links, both formal and informal, will be crucial to this exercise.

The consortia's responsibility to advise on medical education requirements will mean speaking to new 'team players', and this will need to be handled carefully. It will be important to remember that it is the provision of care as a whole that will be important, with the focus centring on the need for the education and training activity, not the separate needs of the various competing professional groups.

Discussion

General considerations

It is important for professionals to understand the general principles of this chapter, and to think about them in relation to their own area of work. It will be important for professionals to know the names of their own consortia members. It may be that professionals have special and specific knowledge which is not common, and could help the consortia members in their work. There is always the opportunity for influence, and for an additional professional perspective on consortia activity. Remember that all the key players are new to this, and that no one is an expert in this process as yet.

It is not clear what the authority of the REDG will be. Will they respond directly to the chief executive of the RO or to the NHS Executive? Who will they be accountable to? What will happen if the consortia and the REDG get it wrong, and we have too many or too few of some professional groups? With the minimum lead in time of 3–4 years there is the potential for such things to happen.

Consortia could have a difficult time coming to life, everyone involved will have other work to do and other things to think about. Consortia have had a very short time span to get themselves together and into working order and this is set against a rapid change agenda both in the Trusts and at the new ROs. There will be a need not only to develop relationships within Trusts, but a compatible working system from the range of consortia members.

Consortia members will be moving into new territory in that the base of educational provision funded through this mechanism will be expanded. Trusts will be expected to consider business plans as one method of identifying educational need, and the need identified will not necessarily be professionally based. There is the opportunity to look at all education and training needs, not just the narrow band of recorded qualifications identified in WP 10. Trusts will also be expected to advise on medical education and training requirements through the consortia framework.

It will be interesting in the future to see where the money goes, (will annual accounts be published?), how the budget is divided, and what will ultimately be included. It will also be important to think about how other costs will be managed, remembering that WP 10 does not include all costs. There will be staff costs, skill-mix issues to be addressed, an organisation's involvement in education and training, and these all need to be considered within the broad framework outlined here. What about the new players? How will the private sector contribute and bid for future staff? Will social service departments start to fund students on the mental health and learning disabilities programmes? Will GPs and GP fund-holders in particular start thinking about how many health visitors, practice nurses, district nurses they will want in the future and start to not only bid for P2000 students, but take them into their practice to learn the work without requiring a fee first?

Educational considerations

Improved education and training provision should be available within the local community, there should be a focus for education and training which is purpose built, and which supports, where appropriate, multi-disciplinary education and training. There will be, where appropriate, opportunities for team building across natural divides for the benefit of patients and clients.

There will be opportunities for increased utilisation of resources through sharing of common facilities; sharing of costs for the major developments; literature sources, collaborative research, and providing a definite focus for getting research into practice (GRIP) and other research and development activities. Opportunities for providing an environment which facilitates education and training both inside and outside clinical and service areas will be able to be explored. The most exciting development will be the opportunity for providing an education and training provision which is firmly rooted in practice by providing ownership by professional groups of the new arrangements; providing opportunities for skill development and enhancement, and providing a resource which can be utilised by all service colleagues to support patient care developments within a geographical area.

Education and training are the foundation upon which the service of tomorrow will be built. There has been a tendency in the past to view education and training as a luxury, and traditionally this element of the budget was one which was cut in times of difficulty. The new culture of the NHS will benefit from more provision for education and training rather than less.

Any arrangement for education and training needs to be on a part-nership basis. Universities or other education providers cannot provide the range and breadth of educational experience needed in today's NHS without working together with the parts of the NHS which provide service. Education and training in the NHS is very much grounded in practice, there is a strong theory/practice base, which is enriching for both research and education. Service issues and needs must be identified and translated into education and training programmes to meet service need.

Any work which is offered by higher education institutions will need to be fully accredited, on the basis of the credit accumulation and transfer schemes (CATS). This will allow for transferability and currency of any educational experience. This will mean that the mobile workforce employed in the NHS will be able to continue their education and training wherever they are working, on a life-long basis. Additionally there needs to be an acknowledgement that a considerable amount of education and training is happening in the workplace itself. Education and service providers need to be working more closely with one another to exploit this learning opportunity, and to find ways to credibly assess the learning that is taking place. Experiential learning, well managed, is of inestimable value to the NHS.

Professional considerations

What would happen if the Trusts stopped including students of nursing and midwifery in their workforce plans and just considered their workforce needs from a nationally produced professional group? Students would go to university like any other graduate group in society. Would this work? Could this work?

Perhaps one of the most interesting things that could happen with the move to higher education would be that all students would become 100 per cent students on a full bursary. There is a tension in the system which is brought about by the imposition of the 80 per cent education/20 per cent service split for funding nursing students. The notion was that this split would give the Trusts some ownership of the student, in fact in some instances it has done the reverse. There is the potential for some Trusts not to train nurses, and use the 20 per cent for other staffing purposes. This is one of the reasons that the consortia need to work together to identify local needs, needs that will consider community Trusts, GP fund-holders and the local voluntary and private sector.

Education and training for professional programmes is a very complex business, it is a wonder that any education institution would want to take it on. For one thing they need to have some practice partnerships to facilitate the process. This can be at a cost to the service provider, a cost which is not always in the budget and cannot be recouped from contract prices. This could lead to an unstable relationship between education and service.

Some outcomes and opportunities of education and training consortia could include:

- Planning education and training for all staff within a geographical area, something which has not really been done before.
- Funding a different, more responsive approach to education and training, particularly in the area of advanced education and practice.
- Sharing expertise in care development, and the education and training requirements to facilitate those developments.
- Allowing local exchange programmes for practitioners to learn from one another in sharing developments, as a unique educational opportunity.
- Developing locally sensitive education and training programmes in partnership with other health providers and local education providers.

Funding of education and training is becoming firmer and more robust. In that a figure has been put to the activity, people involved in the exercise are more aware of the need to identify and quantify costs. There is less opportunity to move money around without at least a degree of communication and negotiation. The money and the whole process is more visible. There are still large areas of uncertainty, and to a degree a lack of clarity. This should be seen as an opportunity, with professionals especially nurses and midwives working hard to reduce the uncertainty, and where possible providing direction and focus. Nurses and midwives have a long association and experience of working in education and training, and managing this area of work within organisations. There is a positive contribution to be made, the profession should make it wholeheartedly while making sure that this opportunity of managing education and training locally works for the benefit of patients and clients.

Acknowledgement

I am particularly grateful for the support of Mr David Loughton, Chief Executive, Walsgrave Hospitals NHS Trust, Coventry, during the preparation of this chapter.

References

Anon (1991) RHAs to have prime responsibility for funding nurse training. *Health Direct*, March, 6–7.

DoH (1989) *Working for Patients*. Cm 555. HMSO, London.

DoH (1993) *The Challenges for Nursing, and Midwifery in the 21st Century – A Report of the 'Heathrow Debate'*. Department of Health, London.

DoH (1994) *Nursing, Midwifery and Health Visiting Education: A Statement of Strategic Intent*. Department of Health, London.

Drucker, P.F. (1990) *Managing in the Non-Profit Organisation*. Butterworth-Heinemann, London.

Funnell, P. (1995) Exploring the value of interprofessional shared learning. In: *Interprofessional Relations in Health Care*, (eds K. Soothill, L. Mackay & C. Webb). Edward Arnold, London.

Goodwin, L. & Bosanquet, N. (1986) *Nurses and Higher Education: The Costs of Change*. Discussion Paper 13. February 1986. Centre for Health Economics, University of York.

Horder, J. (1995) Interprofessional education for primary health and community care: present state and future needs. In: *Interprofessional Relations in Health Care*, (eds K. Soothill, L. Mackay & C. Webb). Edward Arnold, London.

Jarrold, K. (1994) Inaugural meeting of the H.R. special interest group for health care, meeting, 14 September 1994, National Liberal Club, *The Manpower Society*, London.

National Audit Office (1992) *Nurse Education: Implementation of Project 2000 in England*. HMSO, London.

NHSE (1994a) *Implementation of the Report of the Working Group on Specialist Medical Training – 'Hospital Doctors: Training for the Future'*. EL(94)71. National Health Service Executive, London.

NHSE (1994b) *Managing the New NHS: Functions and Responsibilities in the New NHS*. National Health Service Executive, London.

NHSE (1994c) *Transfer of Education and Training Funding*. EL(94)59. National Health Service Executive, London.

NHSE (1995) *Education and Training in the New NHS*. EL(95)27. National Health Service Executive, London.

Pearn, M. (1995) *Methods and Approaches to Help Create a Learning Organisation*. National Health Service Training Division, Bristol.

Perry, L. (1995) Continuing professional education: luxury or necessity? *Journal of Advanced Nursing*, **21**, 766–71.

SCOPME (1995) *The Work of the Standing Committee on Postgraduate Medical and Dental Education. April 1993 to December 1994*. 5th Report. The Standing Committee on Postgraduate Medical and Dental Education, London.

Senge, P.M. (1990) *The Fifth Discipline: The Art and Practice of the Learning Organisation*. Century Business, London.

UKCC (1995) *Implementation of the UKCC's Standards for Post-Registration Education and Practice (PREP)*. United Kingdom Central Council for Nursing, Midwifery and Health Visiting, London.

8
'Credentialling' in Health Care and its Implications

Sue Lillyman

This chapter is a much needed treatise on the current paperchase evident in attempting to measure and recognise the skills and performance of individuals academically and with respect to acquired knowledge and skills. Ms Lillyman discusses the philosophical and practical difficulties encountered in making meaningful observations and judgements about the variable quality of teaching and learning that takes place in practice, and her thorough review of the available literature on the subject should provide practitioners and managers of all disciplines with a grounding in the refinements urgently required to make sense of the credentialling boom currently being enjoyed by universities, publishers and training agencies. The statutory bodies responsible for overseeing credentialling programmes will also find her observations astute and timely.

Introduction

The system of credentialling of clinical practice is a matter for consideration for all health care managers as they are often responsible for the introduction and implementation of systems that measure competence of the practice performed in their clinical area. This chapter begins to explore the concept of credentialling for the practitioner in health care and its implications for the manager. The largest waged part of the workforce is nursing, the implications may, however, be the same for all practitioners within the health care arena. Within health care practice, competence, accreditation and quality have become well known words and concepts that have been discussed and debated within the nursing literature.

Credentialling relates to the issues of competence and quality of care. It attempts to offer an approach that will allow the individual, manager and organisation to differentiate between the levels of competence, offering a system where the practitioner is measured and accredited for their practice, identified at a given level. At present the methods used for credentialling include certification, accreditation, licensure, education and recognition of practice. The consistency and ability to perform is however, far more difficult to measure and raises questions like: where does the practitioner's competency lie? How is that competency evaluated in relation to the ability to perform? And how is the consistency of performance measured? These issues often involve the health care manager directly in the form of the individual performance review or other models used, or the practitioner through the production of a professional profile for the Post-Registration Education and Practice requirements (UKCC 1990).

This chapter will review four key areas for discussion and debate of credentialling. These are primarily differentiating between the levels of practice, identifying what constitutes a specialist practitioner, and therefore who holds what levels of accountability. Secondly I will examine the models used for the discrimination in practice at present and the relationship between competence and quality of care. Thirdly, the role of management education in the process of credentialling is explored. Finally, I will consider the educational opportunities available for individual practitioners to accredit themselves, or work towards a system of credentialling which reflects their ability to perform consistently at an identified level of practice.

What is credentialling?

In nursing practice individuals are gaining additional knowledge and skills to assist them in becoming specialist practitioners. Credentialling is according to Del Bueno (1993) and Archibold and Bainbridge (1994):

'a method used to licence these individuals to practice at an identified level of competence in both clinical practice and knowledge base and then to be awarded some type of accreditation.'

In contemporary nursing practice there is a greater emphasis on the individual practitioner not only to gain competence to practice, but to maintain that competence and to develop from it. This raises the issue of how to demonstrate the ability to prove competence at a given level consistently.

Through the Post-Registration Education and Practice (PREP) and the Professional Code of Conduct, the UKCC (1990; 1992) recommends that the individual must maintain competence. This has been reinforced with the introduction of the professional development profile as implemented on 1 April 1995 (UKCC 1990). It states that all individuals who wish to remain on the practising register as a qualified nurse, midwife or health visitor must produce evidence of their ability and competence to practice. This is achieved through the attainment of a set of educational requirements, in the form of five study days, and a requirement for the individual to identify their personal and professional development through practice. The PREP recommendations also provide an opportunity for some individuals to move on to become a specialist practitioner within a given field of practice. The specialist practitioner is defined by the UKCC (1994), as a 'practitioner who exercises higher levels of judgement and discretion in clinical care'.

The method of accrediting these individuals to become specialist practitioners relies at present on the academic standing of the individual, and the performance and consistency of that practice.

These statements require more exploration. Credentialling goes some way to measuring and identifying that performance through education and practice. It may offer a formal credentialling programme for the individual to attain the competence which is grounded in professional practice and it may lead to the position of specialist practitioner. Fitzpatrick *et al.* (1994) notes that performance can be measured more easily than competence and the difficulties lie in distinguishing between the two. The ability to transfer the competency to different situations and maintain consistency in their performance is another area that raises issues which need to be explored in greater detail.

Levels of performance

The qualities, skills and knowledge of a 'good nurse' has altered over the past few decades, as Jones (1994) argues nursing has responded to the shifts in social and economic conditions moving nursing from a medical to holistic model of care. This shift has brought with it discourse on the professional autonomy and accountability of the individual practitioner. Nurse education has also developed in order to provide a more academic preparation for registration with the move to diploma and baccalaureate programmes. This approach in education assumes that theory precedes practice and as such theory can be applied to the clinical situation.

However, there has been much debate in the nursing literature over the past few decades relating to the theory/practice gap caused in these programmes. There are those who believe there is such a gap (Wong 1979; McFarlane 1986; Kim 1993; Howkins 1994) and those who do not. Dale (1994), for example, argues that the theory is *based* upon practice and the gap is not a theory/practice gap but a theory/theory gap, which she states is evidenced by the apparent lack of experiential knowledge. Jarvis (1994) argues that theory and practice have a dynamic relationship within which practice may at some time precede theory. This has direct relevance to competence. If we accept Jarvis' stance then individuals may need to practice before they reach the required level of performance.

As nursing and midwifery education moves away from the certificate level of the registered nurse qualification to the diploma level of the Project 2000 programme and toward higher academic levels, the relationship between competence accreditation, performance and quality of care will require further discussion and clarification. For example, if the individual studies at a different level is there then an issue of their ability to perform at different levels? Patterson and Haddad (1992) state that nurses practice at different levels of expertise regardless of their education, speciality area or level of care setting.

Carper (1978) notes three types of knowledge, these she refers to as scientific knowledge, personal knowledge and aesthetic knowledge. Burnard (1989) argues that the pre-registration course for practitioners only assists the individual in attaining the first two levels of knowledge, however he argues that the aesthetic, or what he refers to as the 'experiential knowledge', is fundamental to the individual gaining a clear understanding of the meaning of the activity they perform. Mozingo *et al.* (1995) state that the *development of competency* begins with the acquisition of knowledge and skills in the pre-registration education. Traditionally nursing practice has been dependent on the medical model that has been rooted in scientific model and philosophy. Carper (1978) questions 'is it the science of nursing that makes the art possible?' This in turn then leads us to question how the art is to be acquired and then applied into practice?

Tacit knowledge, as described by Meerabeau (1992), identifies the knowing of something only by relying on an awareness of the knowledge to a second activity. This knowledge she then suggests is of a qualitative type, making it difficult to analyse and measure. If this is the situation, how do we measure the individual with a wealth of experiential knowledge who has not gained the recognised qualification? Elliot (1993) states that theoretical abstraction plays a subordinated role in the development of practical wisdom which is then grounded in reflective experiences of concrete cases. However, theoretical analysis does not become dissociated from reality, but is required to gain the experiential knowledge. The factual and practical knowledge is fundamental in the development of the individual understanding the experience or activity.

When this is used to measure competence and award a formal credentialling process it addresses all the levels of knowledge required to identify ability and competence to practice nursing.

The knowledge that the individual gains through their education and training is often measured through the qualification that they hold. To explore this in relation to credentialling we have to go further, to recognise and acknowledge the personal knowledge that has been brought about by experience. This can often discriminate informally between the novice, competent and expert practitioner, as described by Benner (1984). If we look at a practitioner who holds a degree qualification and has therefore proved competent in the academic context, they may still have little experience and only be at the beginner or novice level within a clinical environment. A traditionally registered individual, with no proven academic standing above certificate level may prove themselves to be an expert within the arena of professional practice. However, as Jarvis (1994) notes, the individual who remains in practice does not automatically gain that knowledge and cannot therefore be classed as an expert practitioner merely through time spent in clinical practice.

The problem arising from producing a credentialling programme lies in the required acknowledgement of all the underpinning knowledge bases, recognition of that knowledge, a tool or process to measure the competence that underpins the performance, and a method that identifies consistency in both competence and performance. *Consistency of competence* raises other issues and, as Burnard (1989) notes, the nurses can no longer assume that what they learn today will last for any length of time. Other factors which may affect the level of competency, according to Mozingo *et al.* (1995), is the individual's self-esteem, level of anxiety, stress, previous academic experiences, demographic characteristics and the availability of a good role model for the individual practitioner.

Models of discrimination

There are several models available within the health care arena which attempt to measure the competence level of the individual practitioner within their clinical environment. These have been used in order to identify the human resources that are available and can be utilised within the workplace. They are usually identified by managers as a planning process against a minimum staffing level requirement. These models include the measuring of the academic abilities of the individual, observational studies of the skills performed, patient/client dependency levels, workforce planning and clinical grading. Each approach is used in various areas of practice in an attempt to identify and measure the skills of the practitioner against the perceived needs of the consumer to achieve a high quality of care. There is, however, no reliable method of discrimination and each model will now be reviewed separately.

Academic levels

In nurse education there has been a move to make the practitioner a more 'knowledgeable doer', able to marshal information, make assessments of needs, devise plans of care, and monitor and evaluate them (UKCC 1987). Traditionally nurse education has followed the path of the behaviourist outcomes as described by Pashley and Henry (1990). Training and education took the form of an apprenticeship and the emphasis was firmly on the bio-medical model. There is now an attempt to change this approach with many practitioners now pursuing further education and training in their subject speciality.

The academic model bases its criteria on the measuring of the scientific knowledge of the practitioner. As it stands it possesses quality criteria to which it sets standards and these relate to the academic level of the individual. As in Bloom's (1964) taxonomy, there is a hierarchy of levels of competence ranging from description through to evaluation, and the individual has to attain the level within a given time period. This knowledge base is measured in the qualifications or certificates that the individual has been able to attain. This implies that improving the knowledge base improves the quality of care given. However, Paul and Healsip (1995) state that too much theory content can make it superficial, which results in learning that is only temporary and that therefore we must be aware of the theoretical input to these programmes.

Nursing and midwifery practices are dependent on accurate learning and retention. Dewing (1990) argues that there is no guarantee that the knowledge gained is transferred into the clinical practice. He also states that the complexities of clinical practice are not always possible to solve through the knowledge that originates from academic theory. Just because individuals have completed a course, Burnard (1989) questions whether this is sufficient and suggests that they may not be adequately prepared for all nursing situations. Knowles (1990) views it from a different perspective and suggests that more attention is needed for organisational development, rather than the simple focus on the learning of individuals who work within them. Glen (1995) argues that educators must expand their teaching to include teaching the skills that are involved *to think* and that nursing education and practice cannot rely exclusively on programme content. This model, it may be argued, is used as an attempt to identify the professionalism of nursing. Where there is an emphasis on a distinctive domain of knowledge, the theorising may lead to a basis of power for those who hold the theoretical knowledge (Chinn & Jacobs 1987).

Bjørk (1995) notes a danger in the teaching of theories as it may lead to an increased lack of interest in the practical aspect of nursing. Cave (1994) notes the American experience where the increase in higher education has apparently led to the theory/practice gap becoming significantly worse. However, Manual and Sorensens' (1995) study noted that the baccalaureate nurse was preferred by managers as they were thought to be able to identify a more global view of the care required, and possessed a greater ability to assess and plan patient care. So we must ask the question what is professional development? How can we measure it? And is this measurement of academic achievement a true indication of the level of practice that the individual performs in the clinical setting?

Observational studies

There are popular models that focus on the observation of behavioural skills and attempt to formulate a set of performance criteria or competencies that the individual performs. They attempt to measure the psychomotor skill, but fail to identify the underlying competency that underpins the performance. Based on explicit behavioural or outcome statements they are sometimes referred to as *criterion referenced*. The purpose of this assessment model is to demonstrate an ability to perform specific behaviours within specified standards and within a specific role. They are usually behaviourally based and involve a measurement of an observable behaviour by a third party that can be demonstrated and measured. This model fails to measure the underlying knowledge and competence that the individual has in order to carry out that skill effectively or to consider any bias on the part of the observer.

Johns (1995) notes that becoming an effective practitioner is not simply a question of skills acquisition. Rather it involves a process of personal *deconstruction* and *reconstruction* in dealing with complex situations. It is the tacit knowledge, experiential knowledge, personal and scientific knowledge that all work together to make the practitioner competent in their practice. All of these must therefore be taken into consideration when observing practice. Schön (1987) and Benner (1984) refer to this as the *artistry of practice*; this they state differentiates between the competent and expert practitioner. The question is, how can observable behavioural skills and competencies identify and measure the level of practice that the nurse performs?

What therefore, is the unique role of the qualified nurse? Practitioners themselves find this difficult to articulate. This is relevant in this model in order to help practitioners to identify their competence in practice and the knowledge they require to be able to deliver an acceptable level of care to a specific group of patients/clients. The observational model may attempt to start the process of credentialling the practice. Benner (1984) notes that in the real world of practice there are other issues to take into account such as the ability to make clinical judgments and manage complex situations without relying on formalised rules.

Patient/client dependency models

The National Audit Office in 1985 stated that the requirements for nursing manpower were not always determined systematically by employing authorities to ensure that the numbers employed were fully justified. Together with the introduction of the internal market and the advent of resource managers, other models were implemented to fulfil these requirements. This *patient/client dependency model* is still used in many areas of clinical practice where the perceived dependency of the patient/client is measured using a scoring system and the workforce determined by the results. Gray (1993) notes that demand and supply are not capable of providing an answer to every problem, and nursing operates in areas that are lacking in many of the characteristics of a free market. It is the practitioner's management and psychomotor skills within the therapeutic domain that are measured against the patient/client's level of dependency on the practitioner or the level of bed occupancy.

This model is based on the medical model of care and fails to consider the therapeutic relationship between practitioner and client. Many of these models are dependency driven and utilise an aggregated patient scoring system or the bed occupancy level. They operate on minimum staffing levels, and nursing costs. According to Hurst (1993) little attention is given to professional judgement using these models. Problems arise as the models mask the individual differences in the patient/client receiving the care. A patient/client with a low dependency score, who is ambulant and self-caring in their activities of daily living, would be identified as requiring little nursing care. This may not be the actual situation as this individual may have major social or psychological problems that require the time and expertise of the qualified practitioner. The model also fails to take into account the patient's/client's changing condition and does not usually provide a mechanism to respond appropriately to that change. The model is, however, useful in measuring the nursing activities in the recording and assessment of those psychomotor and tangible skills. It does not measure the total knowledge and the underpinning competence that the practitioner has in order to perform those skills.

The patient dependency model is often used to determine the skill-mix of staff that is required within a given working environment. Skill-mix, argues Wynne (1995), must be distinguished from grade-mix; skill-mix refers to the skill and experience of the individual practitioner *within their grade*. The introduction of this practice Wynne argues is an attempt by management to provide expensive human resources in a more cost-effective way.

This raises the issue relating to the impact that this has on the quality of nursing care given. Skill-mix measures the input and process of nursing, it fails to assess patient outcomes and the quality of patient care (Carr-Hill *et al.* 1992). Bond and Thomas (1991) in their study, raised professional issues relating to this approach. In order to measure accurately there is a need to separate the nursing inputs from the other professional groups, and incorporate individual patients' perceptions to obtain this measurement. Higgins and Dixon (1992) note the failure to take into account the effect of the experience or grade in relation to the organisation of care. McKenna (1995) identified through the literature that managers were often viewed as being more interested in the cost and not the quality, and professionals in the quality not the cost. He argues that this is a simplistic view, as quality is difficult to measure and often invisible to the naked eye. The skill-mix should then reflect the statements and standards of qualified suitable practitioners that are able to perform competently at a designated level in order to achieve appropriate patient/client outcomes and provide quality of care. The question relating to this model of discrimination includes: who decides what nursing is and the way it is to be managed? (Wynne, 1995).

Clinical grading

Clinical grading policy here in the UK emphasised the need to reward 'clinical practice' (Gavin 1995). A pay scale was introduced that rewarded the practitioner for the managerial responsibilities, but did not acknowledge the accrued clinical expertise of the individual (Benner & Tanner 1987). Many individuals were graded according to qualifications as this was an easier process than analysing the job being done by every single nurse. In turn this led to many appeals against grading being upheld. However, the change in resources has since led to many clinical experts or specialist practitioners taking up lower grades to keep their careers (Gavin 1995).

The issue of the specialist and advanced practitioner is now becoming a central debate within the health care arena. This involves a further model of discrimination in the credentialling system that may be related to the grading scale. Holyoake (1995) notes that whilst primary and specialist practice causes little confusion for the practitioner, the UKCC (1994) paper states that the *specialist practitioner* will demonstrate higher levels of clinical decision-making, and monitor and improve standards of care. The level of *advanced practitioner*, he argues, is not so well defined. The UKCC (1995) identifies four main components for the advanced practitioner: these relate to research, education, management and expert practice. Again the question that arises with both the specialist and advanced practitioner is, how is the underpinning competence measured in all these activities and how do we identify and credit 'expert practice'? Benner (1984) argues that this expert practice may not be captured by criteria performance evaluation as already discussed.

Butterworth and Bishop (1995) state that the optimum practice is linked with matters of quality and standards of care. Redfern (1993) in her paper explores the elusive and complex concept of quality of care while Redfern and Norman (1990) note the lack of consistency in the literature of the definition of quality. This measurement therefore is difficult to start to measure if there is no agreed definition (see Chapter 4).

Practitioners are increasingly urged to demonstrate the value of nursing in terms of its effects on the nursing care (Bond & Thomas 1991). However, until nurses can successfully articulate their role and talk in a language that describes their practice, these models and others like them may be used to discriminate the levels and abilities of practice in the clinical situation and credentialling will continue to be awarded on the models.

The role of management and education

For the practitioner the process of continuing education, professional development and life-long learning has become part of maintaining and enhancing knowledge, expertise and competence throughout the individual's career (Hinchliff 1995). This process was highlighted in the government's *Working for Patients* report (DoH 1989) where the quality of training was discussed. A move of nurse education into higher education followed this report. To fulfil the recommendations of the report both education and management have their own roles to play in the continuing education and professional development of the practitioner. Nurse education had until this stage taken place in the college of nursing, it is now acknowledged that learning in the workplace has become the responsibility of management. Both education and management need to work collaboratively in order to develop and provide a system of credentialling that practitioners can achieve and use to prove their competence in performance and practice in the clinical area, which incorporates elements from the cognitive, affective and psychomotor domain. The competence on performance should be transferable to a variety of care situations.

Management

At present the nurse management approach, argues Cowley (1995), is rational, hierarchical and directed primarily at their identified goals. They appear to be governed by objective notions of reliability and predictability. Nurse management is itself having to incorporate a competency based approach, therefore there is a need for competency based learning which will require nurse managers to demonstrate appropriate knowledge and theory of management in their practice (Mulholland 1994). It can be argued that nurses are themselves accountable for their care and as such have a managerial responsibility for the care they deliver to their individual patients/clients. This area needs reviewing from the different levels of practice within it.

The management's responsibility in the role of credentialling performance needs to be reviewed from a variety of perspectives which include: the responsibility to provide opportunities for their employees or subordinates to develop their competency and to provide a reliable means to assess the same, to maintain and improve their own level of competence in the practice of their managerial skills, accountability, and the quality of patient care that is given, and, at whatever level of practice the individual is performing in their managerial role, to assist and support their professional development.

The role of management in education relates to two areas of care. This includes the accountability of the individual practitioner and the quality of care that is administered within the unit or department. Both these areas have an effect on the manager's perceptions of 'credentialling' the individual practitioner in their performance. Health care management has for some time had a commitment to the development of the knowledge base and the accountability of the individual practitioner. As has previously been identified, that theory must not be at the expense of experiential knowledge, which Burnard (1989) states is fundamental to the practitioner in developing a clear understanding of the meaning of the activity they are engaged in. With regard to accountability, the practitioner can only achieve this through analysing the application of the aesthetic knowledge within the context of the experience. Theory and documentation, through the implementation of the nursing process and the named nurse, have increased and provided the base for administration control and accountability. This model of documentation, however, does not reflect the quality of care that the individual or team are providing, but merely measures the quality and ability of record keeping.

Measuring quality of care in nursing has produced a variety of approaches. These include: standard setting, monitor, senior monitor, qualpac, quality circles, audit, independent performance review, quality assurance, etc. Each has been taken, adapted and applied to a variety of clinical environments. The process has attempted to measure the outcomes of the performance in a perceived and measured 'quality' of care given. When asking the patient's view of quality, Webb and Hope (1995) found that, although patients/clients wish to benefit from the information and teaching of the practitioners, they found the patients identified the need for nurses to be more sensitive to the individual patient's opinions and that innovations need to respect the patient's wishes. If this is quality of care then this will have to play a part in the credentialling process in order to integrate theory and practice.

The measurement of competence in practice and the underpinning knowledge base is not taken into consideration for most models of credentialling, although they do go some way to providing some conceptualisation of quality and attempt to measure the actual care, again failing to grasp the totality of the practice performed. Through all of these existing models it is the role of both management and the individual practitioner to protect the patient/client and the individuals working within the environment. The organisation has a responsibility to maintain and develop competence in practice and to acknowledge the level of that practice. As managers prepare to take an active role in professional education they need, argues Cowley (1995), to consider their organisational arrangements and decide how they can assist with learning in the workplace.

Griffiths (1984) introduced the general management structure, and the emphasis on being able to manage rather than administer was introduced. With the NHS reforms (DoH 1989) the market place was also introduced and the manager's role changed accordingly. The ability to manage staff resources and budgets became an essential requirement for those designated as managers. The ward sister/charge nurse, specialist and advanced practitioner are now seen as management positions and as a result have to take on board these management roles.

Programmes of education for the preparation of the management role need to be relevant, realistic, and responsive to their needs (Mulholland 1994).

These management programmes raise the same questions identified in the previous section, how can the competency of the practice of management and the performance be measured in the light of the knowledge and skills that underpin the activity? In Johnson's (1987) study, he identified two types of job competencies: the discriminating competencies that identify the level of performance, and the core competencies that are required to continue with the present job.

Nursing education

With the move of nursing education into higher education we need to ask what this will mean for the practitioners and their patients/clients and the impact if any it will have on credentialling practice. Practitioners must not, argued Glen (1995), fall victim to what she refers to as the 'academic drift' as this will only enhance the theory/practice dichotomy.

Cleverly (1995) argues that nurse education is responsible to society as it uses state financed resources, it is required to be cost effective as well as maintain academic standards. Jarvis (1987) identifies the need for the education process to produce life-long education and that this in turn is important to the quality of performance that they give (Jarvis 1992).

The *Code of Professional Practice* (UKCC 1992) states that:

'just as practice must remain dynamic, sensitive, relevant and responsive to the needs of the patients and clients, so must education for practice.'

With the integration into higher education, Squires (1990) notes that there is a danger that practitioners can have their heads filled with jargon and will no longer be prepared for the real world.

Clarke (1986) and Schön (1987) identify the problems relating to the differences between reality and the ideal. This issue must be taken into consideration with credentialling and practitioners who hold academic qualifications must be able to demonstrate the ability to relate theory to practice and so be competent in the knowledge that underpins performance at all levels of practice. For this reason, states Cleverly (1995), education must evaluate its process effectively; checking for defects at the end of the programme is too slow and too late to prevent poor quality that may in turn affect others within the health care arena.

Education is also attempting to identify what constitutes credibility of the nurse teacher in the higher education scenario. How do they, or do they need to, possess clinical credibility? How do they measure that credibility in relation to the role of educator and the need for them to be aware of the clinical realities that affect the application of theory they teach? And who measures that competence and credibility of practice? The Department of Health in its strategy for nursing (DoH 1989) identified the need for teachers to be 'clinically credible' and the English National Board (1993) stated that 20 per cent of the teacher's time should be engaged in clinical practice. The level of that credibility and competence had led to much debate about the future role of the nurse teacher. Cave (1994) identifies other roles that have affected the education; these include the lecturer practitioner and the link tutor. These roles have been implemented into practice to assist the practitioner with the application of the theory into practice. The issue of practice into theory however has had little debate. Academic qualifications cannot on their own be a basis for a credentialling programme.

Educational opportunities

With the move of nurse education into higher education establishments there have been radical changes and new opportunities for the practitioner in clinical practice. Pashley and Henry (1990) note that these changes will affect the development and enhancement of the clinical role and will change that role for the practitioner. With the general growth of knowledge, research and new technology in all areas of health care, Hinchliff (1994) argues that old skills and knowledge are no longer appropriate. The introduction of the PREP (UKCC 1990) recommendations for nurses, midwives and health visitors has also raised issues concerning the maintaining and developing of professional competence in practice. With the Project 2000 course the level of the basic training has increased to produce a diplomate practitioner and with it there has been an increase in the first level practitioners attaining higher levels of education.

There are a variety of courses on the market at this present time. These range from BTEC to higher degree level courses; all state they prepare the practitioner for their role in practice. BTEC offers courses at the pre-vocational, vocational and continuing education levels and are usually at national, higher national certificate or diploma level. The university system ranges from diploma to higher degree courses. Davis and Burnard (1992) discuss the difficulties in differentiating between diploma, degree, masters, PhD and the 'higher' higher degrees and the route that the individual takes through them. There has been much debate in the quality of the education individuals receive in comparing those who have worked up through the system and those that have omitted one or more level of study, i.e. from diploma to masters or PhD in one move. Davis and Burnard (1992) question whether 'advanced learning' has a direct relationship with 'time spent studying'. This has implications for the practitioner who wishes to access these courses and gain further qualifications.

PREP (UKCC 1990) identifies other issues for all practitioners in that they must produce a profile that demonstrates their professional development and competency in practice through the attendance of five study days, or the equivalent evidence of professional learning. Hogston (1993) notes that this period of study cannot guarantee a change in performance. Davis and Burnard (1992) suggest that this method of education and development are simply seen as a linear process in which learning and experience are accumulated and totted up in some way. Reflective practice has been identified as a process to overcome this situation. Hogston (1993) notes that reflective practice may be based on a sound knowledge and presents a flexible approach to problem solving; it also presents a nebulous quality indicator, however, and again would be problematic in measuring and identifying competence in practice.

If care is central to the practitioner's role, Henry and Pashley (1989) suggest that a qualitative rather than a quantitative approach be used as this may be more suitable and appropriate for the enhancement of health care knowledge. Research that practitioners undertake must also be functional and applicable to practice, incorporating an interdisciplinary approach if practice is to incorporate the underpinning competency, thus affecting and enhancing practice. Post-registration education must take account of these issues and practitioners must be aware of the level and value, both to themselves and to their practice, of the content and application of the course when starting a programme of study.

Conclusion

In conclusion it may be argued that a more structured and valid system is now required to identify what competence in clinical practice is before a system of credentialling can be incorporated. Benner (1982), when assessing clinical competence, states that it should be done in the context of the 'real situation'. As discussed there are difficulties in finding a tool that gives an accurate measurement of competency, or that identifies what the practitioner requires in the way of knowledge to perform safely and effectively in practice. A credentialling system can then be introduced and used in clinical practice that recognises and awards the practitioner for their contribution to a quality service. In my view the models and tools available at present all fail to measure the underpinning competence that makes the unique role of the practitioner. Girot

(1993) notes that there is a potential conflict of the profession's responsibility to produce safe practice. This may lie primarily in the identification of what constitutes competency in practice. The approaches to credentialling that assess the functional aspects of the job do not analyse or consider the demands of the total situation it is attempting to measure (Benner 1982). Watson (1991) argues that the measurement of experience in quantitative terms is widespread, as identified here, however he argues that qualitative measurements are less understood but could be more important in providing this system for the patient/ client, practitioner and organisation.

References

Archibold, P. & Bainbridge, D. (1994) Capacity and competence: nurse credentialling and privileging. *Nursing Management*, **25**(4), 49–56.

Benner, P. (1982) Issues in competency based testing. *Nursing Outlook*, **30**, May, 303–309.

Benner, P. (1984) *From Novice to Expert: Excellence and Power in Clinical Nursing*. Addison Wesley, Menlo Park, CA.

Benner, P. & Tanner, C. (1987) How expert nurses use intuition. *American Journal of Nursing*, **87**(1), 23–31.

Bjørk, I.T. (1995) Neglected conflicts in discipline of nursing. Perceptions of the importance and value of practical skills, *Nursing Times*, **86**(3), 45–6.

Bloom, B. (1964) *Taxonomy of Educational Objectives*. Longman, London.

Bond, S. & Thomas, L. (1991) Issues in measuring outcomes of nursing. *Journal of Advanced Nursing*, **16**, 1492–502.

Burnard, P. (1989) Developing critical ability in nurse education. *Nurse Education Today*, **9**, 271–5.

Butterworth, T. & Bishop, V. (1995) Identifying the characteristics of optimum practice: findings from a survey of practice experts in nursing, midwifery and health visiting. *Journal of Advanced Nursing*, **22**, 24–32.

Carper, B. (1978) Fundamental patterns of knowing. *Advances in Nursing Science*, **1**, 13–23.

Carr-Hill, R., Dixon, P., Gibbs, I., Griffiths, M., McCoughan, D. & Wright, K. (1992) *Skill Mix and the Effectiveness of Nursing Care*. Centre of Health Economics, York University, York.

Cave, I. (1994) Nurse teachers in higher education, without clinical competence do they have a future? *Nurse Education Today*, **14**, 394–9.

Chinn, P. & Jacob, S. (1987) *Theory and Nursing: A Systematic Approach*, 2nd edn. Mosby, St. Louis, MO.

Clarke, M. (1986) Action and reflection: practice and theory in nursing. *Journal of Advanced Nursing*, **11**(1), 3–11.

Cleverly, D. (1995) Quality assurance systems for nurse educators. *Nurse Education Today*, **15**, 303–11.

Cowley, S. (1995) Professional development and change in a learning organisation. *Journal of Advanced Nursing*, **21**, 965–74.

Dale, A. (1994) The theory–theory gap. The challenge for nurse teachers. *Journal of Advanced Nursing*, **20**, 521–4.

Davis, B. & Burnard, P. (1992) Academic levels in nursing. *Journal of Advanced Nursing*, **17**, 1395–400.

Del Bueno, D. (1993) Competence, criteria and credentialling. *Journal of Nursing Administration*, **23**(5), 7–8.

Dewing, J. (1990) Reflective practice. *Senior Nurse*, **10**(10), 26–8.

DoH (1989) *Working for Patients*. Cm 555. HMSO, London.

Elliot, J. (1993) *Action Research for Educational Changes*. Open University Press, Milton Keynes.

English National Board (1993) *Regulations and Guidelines for Approval of Institutions and Courses*. English National Board, London.

Fitzpatrick, J., While, A. & Roberts, J. (1994) The measurement of nurse performance and its differentiation by course preparation. *Journal of Advanced Nursing*, **20**, 761–8.

Gavin, J.N. (1995) The politics of nursing: a case study – clinical grading. *Journal of Advanced Nursing*, **22**, 379–85.

Girot, E. (1993) Assessment of competence in clinical practice: a review of the literature. *Nurse Education Today*, **13**, 83–90.

Glen, S. (1995) Developing critical thinking in higher education. *Nurse Education Today*, **15**, 170–76.

Gray, A. (1993) Defining health needs and the need for nursing. In: *Nursing, Art and Science*, (ed. A. Kitson). Chapman & Hall, London.

Griffiths, P. (1984) Progress in measuring nursing outcomes. *Journal of Advanced Nursing*, **21**, 1092–110.

Henry, C. & Pashley, G. (1989) Vital links. *Nursing Times*, **83**(27), 70–71.

Higgins, M. & Dixon, P. (1992) Skill mix and effectiveness of nursing. *Nursing Standard*, **7**(4), 18–21.

Hinchliff, S. (1994) Learning for life. *Nursing Standard*, **8**, 20–21.

Hinchliff, S. (1995) Practice makes perfect. *Nursing Standard*, **9**(15), 42–3.

Hogston, R. (1993) From competent novice to competent expert: a discussion of competence in the light of the Post-Registration and Education Practice Project (PREPP). *Nurse Education Today*, **13**, 167–71.

Holyoake, D. (1995) Advancing in confusion. *Nursing Standard*, **9**(51), 56.

Howkins, E. (1994) The theory practice gap: can it be closed? *Nursing Standard*, **9**(7), 39–41.

Hurst, K. (1993) *Nursing Workforce Planning*. Longman, Essex.

Jarvis, P. (1987) Life long education and its relevance to nursing. *Nurse Education Today*, **7**, 49–55.

Jarvis, P. (1992) Quality in practice: the role of education. *Nurse Education Today*, **12**, 3–10.

Jarvis, P. (1994) Learning practical knowledge. *Journal of Further and Higher Education*, **18**(1), 31–43.

Johns, C. (1995) The value of reflective practice for nursing. *Journal of Clinical Nursing*, **4**, 23–30.

Johnson, J. (1987) *Job Competency Model.* NHS Training Authority.

Jones, L. (1994) *The Social Context of Health and Health Work.* Macmillan, London.

Kim, H.S. (1993) Putting theory into practice: problems and prospects. *Journal of Advanced Nursing,* **18,** 1632–9.

Knowles, M. (1990) *Adult Learner: A Neglected Species,* 4th edn. GWP Publishers Co., Houston, TX.

McFarlane, J. (1986) The value of models of care. In: *Models of Nursing,* (eds B. Kershaw & J. Salvage, pp. 1–6). John Wiley & Sons, Chichester.

McKenna, H. (1995) Nursing skill mix substitutes and quality of care: an exploration of assumptions from the research literature. *Journal of Advanced Nursing,* **21,** 452–9.

Manuel, P. & Sorensens, L. (1995) Changing trends in health care: education, practice and employment. *Journal of Nursing Education,* **34**(6), 248–53.

Meerabeau, L. (1992) Tacit nursing knowledge: an untapped resource or a methodological headache? *Journal of Advanced Nursing,* **17,** 108–12.

Mozingo, J., Thomas, S. & Brooks, E. (1995) Factors associated with perceived competency levels of graduating seniors in baccalureate nursing program. *Journal of Nursing Education,* **34**(3), 115–22.

Mulholland, J. (1994) Competency based learning applied to nursing management. *Journal of Nursing Management,* **2,** 161–6.

National Audit Office (1985) *Report by the Comptroller and Auditor General: NHS Control of Nursing Manpower.* HMSO, London.

Pashley, G. & Henry, C. (1990) Carving out the nursing nineties, *Nursing Times,* **86**(3), 45–6.

Patterson, C. & Haddad, B. (1992) The advanced nurse practitioner: common attributes. *Canadian Journal of Nursing Administration,* **5**(4), 18–22.

Paul, R. and Healsip, P. (1995) Critical thinking and intuitive nursing. *Journal of Advanced Nursing,* **22,** 40–47.

Redfern, S. (1993) In pursuit of quality of nursing care. *Journal of Clinical Nursing,* **2,** 141–8.

Redfern, S. & Norman, I. (1990) Measuring the quality of nursing care: a consideration of different approaches. *Journal of Advanced Nursing,* **15,** 1260–71.

Schön, D. (1987) *Educating the reflective practitioner.* Jossey Bass, San Francisco, CA.

Squires, G. (1990) *First Degree: The Undergraduate Curriculum.* Open University Press, Milton Keynes.

UKCC (1987) *The Final Proposals, Project Paper 9.* United Kingdom Central Council for Nursing, Midwifery and Health Visiting, London.

UKCC (1990) *The Report of Post-Registration, Education and Practice Project (PREPP report).* United Kingdom Central Council for Nursing, Midwifery and Health Visiting, London.

UKCC (1992) *Code of Professional Conduct.* United Kingdom Central Council for Nursing, Midwifery and Health Visiting, London.

UKCC (1994) *The Future of Professional Practice. The Council's standards for Education and Practice Following Registration.* United Kingdom Central Council for Nursing, Midwifery and Health Visiting, London.

UKCC (1995) *Post-Registration Education and Practice*. United Kingdom Central Council for Nursing, Midwifery and Health Visiting, London.

Watson, S. (1991) An analysis of the concept of experience. *Journal of Advanced Nursing*, **16**, 1117–21.

Webb, C. & Hope, K. (1995) What kind of nurses do patients want? *Journal of Clinical Nursing*, **4**, 101–108.

Wong, J. (1979) The inability to transfer classroom learning into clinical nursing practice. *Journal of Advanced Nursing*, **4**, 161–8.

Wynne, T. (1995) Skill mix in nursing: efficiency and quality. *Journal of Nursing Management*, **3**, 189–91.

Part IV
MANAGING PARADOX

9
The Politics of Health Care
Alison Morton-Cooper

This final chapter of the book is intended to provide a wide-ranging review of the broader and increasingly global macro-economic and political issues affecting the distribution and outcomes of health care interventions. The contradictions apparent within formalised state provision and the culturally mediated responses which form ever louder demands for more investment in welfare, technological interventions, health promotion and 'illness care', lie at the heart of this discussion.

Has the rise of managerialism finally succeeded in abating the onslaught of medical dominance and power, or are we, as ever, beholden to recognised 'health professionals' for the proper and legitimate determination of need within populations and communities? What are the political undercurrents facing managers in their everyday attempts to manage effectively and efficiently in the best interests of patients and clients? And whose best interests does the continuing technological revolution in diagnosis and treatments serve? In short, what has medical science ever done for us?

What does the future hold for those who are increasingly becoming mere spectators in the struggle to achieve health for all within a health care bureaucracy facing spiralling costs and a depersonalisation of the art of caring? Using paradox as a method of critical analysis, what amounts to a fair criticism of current provision, and what alternative strategies can we devise for recognising and rewarding excellence in health care? Given the current ideological 'propaganda battle for the allegiances of the people' here in the UK (Butler 1992), who will be brave enough to confront the anomaly of increasing health care output leading to even greater demand on an already overstretched health care system? Much depends, as Butler says, on how you view recent British NHS reforms. Have they left the NHS as 'the unfortunate victim of a mugging that ought never to have occurred'; are they 'an exercise in the blind application of ideology', or, more optimistically, 'the replacement of one set of principles for managing a public service industry with

*another better attuned to the spirit and technologies of the time'?
(Butler 1992, p. 120). What do the public want from their health services, and what indices do we rely on to measure their relative successes? Is interprofessional and collaborative care the answer, and if
so, with whom should we collaborate? The author argues that a heli-
copter perspective on social welfare and on the evolving challenges to
professional dominance is an essential prerequisite in trying to
understand the power relationships in contemporary organisations,
and the contexts in which they claim to function. What are the human
and social costs associated with scientific medicine, and what interests do we have in analysing and quantifying these costs? Whose vested
interests are at stake in continuing to promote technological solutions
to our human and social problems?*

*As managers whose job it is to oil and maintain social and health
services as the recognised 'engine' of the welfare state, the ability to
critically analyse health policy is thus arguably a key skill for health and
social service employers in a modern democracy. The freedom to express
and explore alternative world-views on what constitutes good practice
in health care, unconstrained by anachronistic or patronising conceptions of gender, race and age, is but one aspiration for a service which
claims to provide for a multicultural society. To what extent are health
interventions (ostensibly designed to empower the public) a mechanism
of social control, and how can these be legitimised by the actions and
value systems of health care managers as agents of the state?*

*The purpose of the final part is to open up the debate as to the ideo-
logical determinants of policy debate, so as to create a greater awareness and cognisance of the ways in which debate within health care is
inextricably linked to the wider issues of politics, economy and philosophical understanding of what constitutes good health in a post-
modern society.*

Introduction

Charles Handy's work (1994) *The Empty Raincoat: Making Sense of the
Future* offers a striking contemporary metaphor in its frank discussion of
the many paradoxes or apparent self-contradictions afflicting our planet
as it veers headlong towards a new millennium. Handy says he no longer
believes in the 'theory of everything', or in the possibility of perfection.

'Paradox I now see is inevitable, endemic and perpetual. The more
turbulent the times, the more complex the world, the more the paradoxes.'

(Handy 1994, p. 17)

He is pessimistic of our collective abilities to dissolve or resolve the 'puzzles in the paradoxes'. Like the weather, we have to live with them and enjoy them as best we can. Living with them won't be comfortable or easy, but if we are to make some kind of sense of our future, then

'paradox has to be accepted, coped with and made sense of, in life, in work, in community and among the nations.'

(Handy 1994, p. 18)

It is therefore in suitably Handyesque form that I dedicate this section of the book to an examination (personal though it may be) of some of the prevailing paradoxes apparent in health care and its management.

The meaning of paradox

Personally, I find it easier to view paradox as an absurdity – the reverse of what you would expect to be true. In this part of the book my theme is essentially an exploration of the ways in which the study of paradox can help to explain and demystify some of the apparent contradictions in the provision and management of health care.

paradox: a statement or tenet contrary to received opinion or belief; a statement seemingly self-contradictory or absurd, though possibly well-founded or essentially true.

(Oxford English Dictionary)

thesaurus alternatives to paradox: conflicting, enigma, mystery, puzzle, quandary, dilemma, absurdity, problem.

(Oxford Thesaurus)

The origins of modern health and welfare systems

No discussion of contemporary health care would be complete without at least an overview of earlier conceptions of health and healing. As a starting point, the medical historian Katherine Park describes the care offered to the population of medieval Europe:

'Doctors became monks and monks, doctors. Lay healers treated the religious, and the religious, the laity. Magic played a part in the natural medicine of both rich and poor.'

(Park 1992, p. 70)

Medieval conceptions of healing considered it a craft rather than an intellectual discipline.

Until the introduction of formal standards for training and apprenticeships and set medical curricula in the twelfth century, little was really known about the nitty gritty of practice:

'What little was known of the healers who worked in the courts, monasteries and villages points to an inclusive system of medicine, where a variety of practitioners – clerical and lay, male and female, literate and illiterate – and a variety of approaches to healing co-existed in loose relationships of co-operation and competition.'

(Park 1992, p. 70)

The fifteenth century saw the introduction of systematic dissection of the human body and the production of anatomical atlases, such as those created by Vesalius (*De Humani Corporis Fabrica* 1543). This allowed the body to be represented three-dimensionally allowing the differentiation of internal and external body structures, so that an observer was able to 'view' internal organs from the outside without dissection, constituting notable progress on earlier methods (Wedding 1995, p. 446). The enthusiasm of the French philosopher René Descartes to establish a direct connection between the body and the soul carried profound implications for our developing perceptions of 'self'. His conceptions of mind–body dualism – the interrelationship between the mechanical functions of the body and the spiritual aspirations of the soul – have served as an influential model for several modern schools of psychology, the most famous of which is probably psychoanalysis (Lundin 1991, p. 40). As Wedding explains:

'From this position Descartes proceeded to argue for the existence of two classes of substance that together constitute the human organism: the palpable body, a product of nature, and the intangible mind, which Descartes claimed God had given to humans so they could examine and understand nature.'

(Wedding 1995, p. 446)

The corollary of this, as far as Wedding is concerned, is that this formulation gradually opened the door to the reductionist approach characteristic of modern science, including medicine and modern medical practice. In the period which came to be known as the Enlightenment he claims that several principles came to be accepted:

'Among them [is] the idea that an objective, scientific approach to diagnosis and therapy is essential.'

(Wedding 1995, p. 446)

Within the next hundred years the expansion of public hospitals was associated with greater social mobility and the growth of towns across

Europe. The consequent immigration of people from rural to developing areas, intensified by the impact of nineteenth century industrialisation, led to a greater density of population and readier access to patients for healers intent on practising their art. Earlier, medieval and individualistic religious notions of illness signifying God's judgement on the sinful (so called 'divine retribution' for sins inherent or committed) came to be displaced by the increasing recognition of specific disease entities which shared common traits, regardless of the individual sufferer:

'Under the new schema, diseases were localised first to the organ, and later to tissue and cell. The focus therefore shifted from the whole body to the diseased part. The emphasis was less on symptoms reported by the patient, now seen as subjective, and more on signs that could (in theory) be objectively measured, often with the use of instruments, by the doctor.'

(Granshaw 1992, p. 204)

The attribution of poor health to structural and environmental factors and causes was still some way off, although the distinctions between the 'deserving poor' and the undeserving so prevalent in Britain in the Victorian era could be said to remain to this day (see Hutton 1995). The adage of cleanliness being next to godliness made spiritual health the business of priests and religious advisers, who were themselves aware of the effects of poor sanitation and damp overcrowded housing on the material conditions of the urban poor (Barker 1995). The explosion in scientific discovery and knowledge about causative agents (the advent of so-called 'germ theory') led to the increasing professionalisation of medicine, and the creation of teaching hospitals and medical schools dedicated to the study of the human body (see Weatherall (1995) for a detailed history).

The very notion of 'expertise' in a subject led to the institutionalisation of the professions. Systems of government came to be linked inexorably to the

'classification and surveillance of populations, the normalisation of the subject-citizen and the discipline of the aberrant subject.'

(Johnson *et al.* 1995, p. 11)

As systems of government developed, critical boundaries of 'normality' were set, and citizens could be classified in relation to governmentally decreed 'norms'.

It was perhaps at this time that notions of deviance and arbitrary distinctions of normality/abnormality came to be recognised and used to assess the characteristics of the population, with subsequent opportunities for the development of 'corrective' government policy. With the benefit of twentieth century hindsight we can see how the governmental systems of public health, formal schooling and a regulated prison service came into being as a collective response to apparent deficiencies in the control of communities and the burgeoning need for purposeful economic development.

Pressures for reform and national efficiency

Here in Britain, social problems emerging from the stealthy advance of industrialisation were eloquently criticised by reformers and philosophers (for example Thomas Carlyle and John Stuart Mill, see Clayre (1977) for an anthologised treatise on the conditions and aspirations of the time), and called for concerted remedy and active reform.

Not least was the demand for 'social efficiency' characterised in a determined opposition to all forms of *waste:*

'the human and fiscal costs of *not* preventing dangers to health, economic performance and national efficiency, had long been the standard argument for state intervention in public health, factory reform, slum clearance, poor law medical treatment, state education, workmen's compensation and the like.'

(Perkins 1989, p. 155)

The potential waste of human resources was seen as the most damaging and divisive, particularly with regard to the working class, who it seemed had little recognisable opportunity to improve their prospects without access to organised forms of education and greater literacy.

The rise of 'welfarism'

Perkins (1989) describes the traditionally accepted 'causes' of the British Liberal welfare measures of Edwardian times as a response to three different kinds of pressure:

- 'pressure from below' arising from the groundswell of political demands from an increasingly vocal working class
- 'pressure from facts' – the impact on public opinion of the new knowledge of poverty and distress documented by leading social reformers and army recruiters of the time
- 'pressure of intolerability' – the extent to which problems were perceived to be a threat to the drive for 'national efficiency'.

Even though fear of the poor and potential uprisings might conceivably have added to the pressure for change, Perkins points out that the arbiters of 'intolerability' were not the revolutionary public, but rather the Oxford idealists, Cambridge welfare economists, Fabian and other middle-class socialists of the time, who emphasised:

'the responsibilities of property, national efficiency and justification by service to society.'

(Perkins 1989, p. 161)

Whatever the intentions or predictions of commentators at the time, a professionally institutionalised system of welfare was the outcome of the reformers' deliberations. The exacerbation of existing social problems brought on by the privations of two world wars led ultimately to the introduction of new pillars of government. The institution of central government departments, elected local authorities and the newly created National Health Service (NHS) were seen as the most effective means of delivering the core services of social security, health care, education and housing, and the personal social and welfare services (Butcher 1995).

Thus the *public administration model of welfare* was born, underpinning the delivery of welfare services from 1945 onwards, and one which came to be the role model for other national governments to challenge or emulate. Butcher has identified the five core characteristics of this model:

- a bureaucratic structure
- professional domination
- accountability to the public
- equity of treatment
- self-sufficiency.

Together, the fast developing professional bureaucracy came to represent a particular philosophy of care provision dedicated to the amelioration of what came to be popularised as 'the five giant evils on the road to reconstruction haunting post-war Britain: want, disease, ignorance, squalor and idleness (Beveridge 1942; Timmins 1995). Whether Beveridge ever envisaged or intended the monolithic creation of the vast numbers of institutions and employees, which have since come to represent British welfarism, is unknown. What is clear, however, is that various forms of professional work came to dominate provision in the mid-twentieth century. Armies of doctors, teachers, social workers and other public servants came to represent the embodiment of welfarism from 'cradle to grave'.

The Paradox of Welfare

The amount of power enjoyed by welfare professionals, and the economic and social consequences of their labours over the last 40 years, have been the subject of many animated debates and controversies as to cost efficiency and have variously been accused of reducing client autonomy, and instead increasing *dependency*, which if it were ever accepted as true, would undoubtedly deserve recognition as the *paradox of welfare*, or what Lewis (1992) has described as *diswelfare*.

According to Butcher (1995), professionals wield their power in the following ways:

• by being able to make and administer policy themselves
• by their accepted right to define the needs and problems of their clients
• by their influence in the allocation of resources (e.g. management of budgets, the development of services and so on)
• by the self-regulation of their professions.

Butcher points out that although historically it has not always been the state's role to both fund and provide services to the public, it increasingly began to do so (Butcher 1995). The interventionist role played by the state in constantly redefining and shaping public policy assured it a central place in the public's collective consciousness in Britain, so much so that the instruments and outcomes of 'welfarism' now constitute a powerful and emotive electoral issue at general and local elections. As George and Wilding have wryly observed:

'intervention grows when politics comes to be dominated by democratic competition for votes.'

(George & Wilding 1994, p. 19).

The concept of need

Jane Lightfoot of the Social Policy Research Unit at the University of York has warned that the definitive meaning of 'need' continues to be elusive, even though consensus on what constitutes need is an essential prerequisite for the effective functioning and collaboration of the recently reformed health and social care agencies. As she points out, if all needs were capable of being met, rigour in defining need would not be so critical (Lightfoot 1995). With greater media attention being devoted to the apparent necessity for rationing limited health resources here in the UK a more open discussion and confrontation regarding the choices open to us would seem to be required. As Lightfoot explains:

'In policy terms, given the possibility of different interpretations of "need", clarity is required about the definition in use, along with criteria for setting priorities. For example, the following questions must be addressed: what is a definition of need? Is there a separation between ends such as a need for health, and means, a need for health services? If so, what definition of "health" is to be used?'

(Lightfoot 1995, p. 108)

Once questions of ethicality and social justice are asked, the debate of course becomes more complex:

'How are priorities set? Is there a hierarchy of needs satisfaction? If so, how is this defined? How is the tension between "economic efficiency" and "social justice" in resource allocation resolved?'

(Lightfoot 1995, p. 108)

Effective interagency and provider collaboration may be the key to providing the care most appropriate to people's needs in contemporary setting, as Lightfoot says, but as she also points out, there is a need to change culture, values and attitudes in favour of a joint approach to care. Recognising that conceptual difficulties will always make pure and uncontested definitions unlikely, she suggests the way forward is through examination of the values and assumptions underpinning professional choices.

The political nature of decisions means that interpretation of needs and priorities on the boundary between health and social care is always likely to remain contested.

'It follows that there are persistent dangers of gaps and overlaps in care arising from misalignments of judgements about need and priorities, both between purchasers and providers in the same agency and between those who operate at agency boundaries. Such dangers serve to reinforce the need to make such judgements explicit.'

(Lightfoot 1995, p. 113)

What this means in reality is that access to services is unlikely to be equitable, and that the ideological crisis over the deserving and the undeserving is set to continue, with welfare professionals wielding as much power as central government permits them to. The ideological battle between supporters of comprehensive, universalist welfare services and those on the New Right who espouse market-led, commercially based solutions looks set to continue indefinitely (Jones 1994).

In fairness, the problem of rationing and its social and economic consequences lies at the heart of all attempts at reform in health care and is an international problem affecting governments of all political hues (see Seedhouse (1995) for a helpful overview of international health reform).

The Paradox of Health Care Provision

What we are left with in the 1990s then, is the *paradox of health care provision*. The more care we provide, the more knowledge we acquire about disease and genetics, the more demand we generate for the professional health and welfare services. As standards of health and living conditions improve for some sections of the community (generally speaking, the already better off), more inequities are identified and thrown into sharp relief. It would seem to follow then that the more professionals we employ to determine needs and priorities, the more justification we can find for spending fiscal resources and time on their possible solutions. It is the sustainability (or otherwise) of this bureaucratic system of welfare which increasingly looks to global solutions for an answer to increasingly global problems. But who should be responsible for a nation's health, and what are the alternatives to the socialist system? (See articles by Schubert-Lehnhardt and Cribb in Seedhouse (1995) for an insightful perspective on the alternatives.) At a more fundamental level, what is this concept of 'health' which underpins our cultural assumptions about care provision, and why as policy-makers and managers is some degree of consensus on the subject necessary to inform policy formation and care delivery?

Health in crisis

The health ethicist David Seedhouse claims that the world of health is in crisis; a crisis caused by our conceptual confusion and muddle over what 'health' actually means. We have, it would seem, lost our sense of what health is. In his view, health has come to be seen as synonymous with *human value*. Health is increasingly regarded as a right extending even beyond birth. He doesn't predict an early or easy solution to our difficulties, but he does offer an insight into their (possible!) root and branch:

'For over 200 years in the western nations, professional health care has been associated almost exclusively with medicine and the medical establishment, but in recent years new trends and forces have emerged as challengers to the traditional order. Some of these pressures have been generated by the dissatisfaction and disquiet of people who have experienced the medical version of health care as outsiders, but many have occurred as a natural consequence of there being theoretical and practical problems that traditional medicine is badly equipped to tackle. Such forces inevitably pose a challenge to the very idea that medicine is and should be the single focus of health care.'

(Seedhouse 1988, p. 3)

Disillusionment with the outcomes of conventional medicine and the spiralling costs of science-based medicine has certainly resulted in some very eloquent and stinging examples of (metaphorical!) doctor-bashing in recent years. Bryan Christie, health correspondent of the *Scotsman* newspaper, has suggested that something like 80 per cent of all medical treatments have never been evaluated fully for effectiveness, although he recognises that full clinical trials are not always practical, necessary of indeed desirable. He suggests as few as 20 per cent of medical treatments are of any proven benefit to patients (Christie 1995a). He bases these claims on a report by Dr William Rosenberg in the *British Medical Journal*, which is reported to have stated:

'We (doctors) continue to base our clinical decisions on increasingly out of date primary training or the overinterpretation of experiences with individual patients and even dramatically positive results from rigorous clinical studies remain largely unapplied.'

(Rosenberg cited in Christie 1995a, p. 15)

The power of doctors has undoubtedly grown as society has declined religion in favour of a more secular approach to human problems:

'The decline of organised religion ... led to doctors being cast more and more in the role of secular priests whose expertise encompassed not only the treatment of bodily ills but also advice on how to live the good life, and judgements on right and wrong.'

(Zola 1972 cited in Gabe *et al.* (1994), p. xii)

As if it weren't enough for us to contemplate the possibility that doctors may not, in fact, be the creditable fount of all wisdom and bodily knowledge, Coward (1989) warns us to beware of the 'cultural blackmail' executed by the 'consciousness industries' of alternative health movements which tempt us with the promise of making us 'whole':

'... in the alternative health movement, this original state of well-being and the one to which all activities aspire, is conceived of as a state balance and harmony. Self-healing is possible if and when this state of balance is restored. And here we confront an apparent paradox. For if the body harbours this impulse towards good health, why should we succumb to illness at all?'

(Coward 1989, p. 51)

The Paradox of Caring

Other distinguished clinicians have rallied to the defence of modern medicine, arguing that there is more to practice than science, but that the overworked doctors of today have little opportunity to take proper account of their impact on individuals and families. In a treatise on the impact of medical research on the evolution of modern medicine, David Weatherall, Regius Professor of Molecular Medicine at the University of Oxford, states a case for doctors today. He argues that young doctors attempt to analyse and treat their patients' illnesses on the basis of their scientific training and knowledge, but occasionally they find themselves with incomplete knowledge. Some form of therapy, even if of unproven value, then has to be tried. As more medical knowledge is acquired:

'the more difficult it is for the critical and caring clinician to dissociate their scientific training from the practical necessity of doing something to relieve suffering, even though they are rarely sure about what they are doing.'

(Weatherall 1995, p. 52)

Doctors still have to live with uncertainty in an uncertain world.

Professor Weatherall charts the progress of medical science from the beginnings of medical instrumentation and early diagnostic aids, to responses to the pandemics affecting the world of tomorrow. Most importantly, he touches on the 'old' clinical virtues of good doctoring:

'Why do they seem to have been lost in our increasingly mechanistic world? Might they become completely redundant as we progress towards a genuine understanding of disease, and as medical practice evolves from an "art" to a "science"?'

His tone is reassuring:

'... there is no fundamental contradiction between the scientific approach to the study and management of disease and the pastoral aspects of medical care. On the contrary, as we develop even more sophisticated patterns of clinical practice, with all the new ethical issues that they will pose, the need to treat patients as people, and not diseases, will be all the greater.'

(Weatherall 1995, p. 22)

This we might describe as the *paradox of caring*. As science continues to depersonalise us, reducing us to genetic matter predisposed to certain afflictions and debilities, the demand for a caring, personalising approach is likely to increase in direct relation to the rise in scientific knowledge. In short, human health care will have to become an 'art' again.

Challenging medicine: health beliefs and doctor power

In order to understand the paradox of caring in more depth, some analysis of the health beliefs informing popular culture and behaviour is perhaps necessary. Sally Thorne has described the cultural components of health belief *systems* (an intriguing notion in itself), as the nature of health, the nature of illness and the role of the healer. Thorne contends that the dominant belief system in the west is that of 'biomedicine' which she believes is powerful enough to have achieved a position of social prominence sufficient to allow it political and legal dominance over all other competing belief systems (Thorne 1993). She stresses the close association of biomedicine with the culture of imperialism of the nineteenth century, and with the major social trends towards scientism, positivism and rationalism (in other words the notion that a recognisable system of natural order can be achieved).

Disease came to have scientific labels, and with the establishment of specific disease categories the main task of diagnosis became one of approximating the patient's pathology to an established disease category through observation, physical examination and the study of various biochemical parameters (Morgan *et al.* 1988). The dominance of scientific medicine resulted in the human body being equated with a machine, with the approach then being allied to promoting health through medical interventions. The interpersonal and socio-environmental models of health intervention (as opposed to the dominant biomedical model) took a back seat to advancing health technologies.

In considering whether scientific medicine serves both the interests of the medical profession and the functional needs of society, Morgan *et al.* refer to the influential work of Ivan Illich, who had lambasted medical bureaucracy and its effects on the population, claiming that by 'duping the public into believing it has an effective and valuable body of knowledge and skills' it had created a dependence of doctors on medicine which had taken away their individual and collective abilities to engage in self-care (Morgan *et al.* 1988, p. 23). Illich claimed that the medical establishment constituted a radical monopoly on health care in society. The insidious and damaging effects of such a dependency created what he called an 'iatrogenesis' (literally *doctor-created*) disease state of both clinical and societal proportions.

A dependent culture then came to define itself in relation to the legitimacy handed down by doctors (and presumably the same could be said of other welfare 'experts', such as nurses, social workers, midwives and so on). Illich's point was uncompromisingly political:

> 'A radical monopoly feeds on itself. Iatrogenic medicine reinforces a morbid society in which social control of the population by the medical system turns into a principal economic activity. It serves to legitimise social arrangements into which many people do not fit. It labels the handicapped as unfit and breeds ever new categories of patients. People who are angered, sickened and impaired by their industrial labor and leisure can escape only into a life under medical supervision and are thereby seduced or disqualified from political struggle for a healthier world.'
>
> (Illich 1976, p. 43)

The intention of health care, ostensibly to empower and improve the life chances of individuals and groups within a community, from this perspective is clearly paradoxical. Continued reliance on the biomedical model is viewed as the outcome of a capitalist/industrial economy: murky discussion territory for aspiring health managers! But Illich takes no prisoners. Rather eerily, he sees twenty years into the future, describing what (for some, at least) has come to pass:

> 'Social iatrogenesis is not yet accepted as a common etiology of disease. If it were recognised that diagnosis often serves as a means of turning political complaints against the stress of growth into demand for more therapies that are just more of its costly and stressful outputs, the industrial system would lose one of its major defenses. At the same time, awareness of the degree to which iatrogenic ill-health is politically communicated would shake the foundations of medical power much more profoundly than any catalogue of medicine's faults.'
>
> (Illich 1976, p. 43)

It could, therefore, be argued that many of the stressful conditions existing in work habits and environments, such as long hours and the need for increased production output, are in fact legitimised by medicine rather than ameliorated by it as we might expect.

Occupational psychology has evolved as a discipline in response to empirical problems of human stress responses, and it is the degree to which personal responsibility can be taken for stress-induced illness (rather than directing it at ill-conceived government policy direction) which continues to tax us in coming to terms with the social construction and veritable existence of 'stress' (see Warr (1987); Newton *et al.* (1995) and Kasl & Cooper (1995) for an enlightening discussion of this emotive topic). The central role played by doctors (including psychiatrists and their colleagues in clinical psychology) is of critical importance in considering the paradox of caring, for it could be argued that it is only when an illness is publicly accepted and legitimated by biomedicine, that the individual comes to be recognised officially by the state welfare machine, their employers, friends and families. This adds up to what could be viewed as the *paradox of control*, whereby individuals who ostensibly stand to be empowered by the services of health and welfare, can equally well be disempowered, if for some reason formal recognition of their 'pathology' is not biomedically acknowledged. Sufferers of repetitive strain injury (RSI) and myalgic encephalomyelitis (ME) are good examples of the struggle necessary to mobilise needed health resources in relation to apparently discernible symptoms requiring formal legitimation.

The wider political and economic consequences of problems arising from the use of modern technologies, or from the physiological and psychological outcomes of contemporary lifestyles, are a huge political concern. Illich for example, might reasonably argue that both are examples of medicine acting as agents of state control. If both 'conditions' were formally recognised, what would the legal and financial implications mean for employers and the major corporations which have grown up with the adoption of new office and information technologies? Paradoxically, formal recognition can also work against the interests of the individual as it may necessitate a withdrawal from productive public life, on terms unconducive to personal autonomy and freedom to act. Turner has pointed out, for example, that there is a further paradox in modern societies, which is that the greater demand for personal equality in provision, the greater the requirement for surveillance and regulation of society:

'The medicalization of society involves a detailed and minute bureaucratic regulation of bodies in the interests of an abstract conception of health as a component of citizenship.'

(Turner 1995, p. 217)

The broader political implications of other definitively recognised conditions are also food for thought. Childhood and occupational asthma sustains a vast pharmaceutical industry, the profits from which, paradoxically, research funds are found. Reluctance to ascribe the epidemic proportions of asthma to vehicle exhaust pollution is arguably because to blame such environmental pollution would require a reversal of trends to sell cars, develop roads and extend private transport and (in theory) undermine the economy on which Britain, and other advanced industrial societies, is largely based.

Several recent conflicting studies on the impact of exhaust pollution have confounded the experts, and led to policy inertia; this, it seems, as a consequence of a lack of political will on the part of central government and the medical lobby to confront the politics of asthma. With the increasing tendency towards litigation for damages, who could contain the potential claims for state welfare benefits and compensation for personal injury brought about by economic growth and the might of the pharmaceutical industries? The legitimacy given by doctors to a particular disease entity can give access to welfare benefits, political ammunition to 'green' lobbyists, greater opportunities for pharmaceutical firms to increase their profits, and ultimately do much to influence the lifestyle and life opportunities of individuals and their families. 'What did the doctor say?' has become a major configuration in people's lives.

There is even the bizarre example of Münchhausen's syndrome, whereby the lonely and distressed are prepared to self-mutilate in order to secure the care and attention of others deprived them by other social means (Feldman & Ford 1994).

Some authors view doctor power as having distinct elements. One is that of a powerful pressure group (so-called 'macro-power'), and the other is in decision-making at an individual level ('micro-power') (Harrison *et al.* 1992). The resource implications of clinically based decisions, it seems, are rarely questioned by health managers, and when they are, doctors are prone to react with indignation and distrust of the manager's motives.

The resulting conflict, and suggestions for ways around this conflict, is discussed in an eye-opening article by Drife and Johnston (1995) who say that the potential for conflict arising from cultural differences is almost limitless. They argue that mutual respect between colleagues is essential, together with an exploration of values, shared objectives and a reduction in what is intriguingly described as 'disinformation':

> 'One way of stimulating frank discussion is to breach etiquette by putting the hidden agenda on the table.'
>
> (Drife & Johnston 1995, p. 1056)

The paradox of control in the pharmaceutical industries is not so easy to address. On the one hand, dependence on research funding from the large corporations leaves a dubious legacy. It is obviously in the short-term interests of corporate business to generate profit from the sale and distribution of medicines, treatments and sophisticated technical equipment. Profits equal taxes which result in income to the state. On the other hand, if we depend on the profits to discern the causes of pathological conditions, the pharmaceutical industry experiences a conflict of interest. Is the best answer to discern and publicise the cause (which may in effect result in some relief from distress), or to respond to the problem with a more sophisticated technicised solution in the form of manufactured drugs or preventive/relieving equipment? The choice is not always clear or straightforward for the public (or indeed the industry) to determine. The problems associated with bovine spongiform encephalitis (BSE) or so-called 'mad cow disease' have, as an example, caused serious concern among farmers, not least because of the potential claims for damages arising from what some perceive as poor advice from central government, but equally from other alleged causes, such as pesticide poisoning and reported human cases of BSE, the neurological condition known as Creutzfeldt-Jakob disease (Christie 1995b).

Whilst it could be argued that all health and welfare professionals have the potential to do damage to individuals and groups through incompetence, overwork or misdiagnosis, it is doctors alone who stand in the cross-fire between central government and industry. So if, as Professor Weatherall says, doctors have to live and work in an uncertain world, it seems we do too.

Beliefs about health and illness are grounded in people's wider understanding of the world we live in, and the place we ascribe to ourselves within it. This means that we draw upon a stock of knowledge about sickness, and about its bodily signs, that owes much to our cultural setting and inheritance (Radley 1994). Critiques which examine, for example, the new reproductive technologies currently developing in health care are quick to highlight the cultural and social predicaments they represent. The paradox of caring can be examined in this context in relation to the impact scientific medicine has had on the lifestyles of western women.

Women and medical power

One of the best documented examples of medical control in society is arguably that of women and the health care industry. Foster (1995), for example, has strongly criticised the impact of new reproductive technologies for its domination over women of all social groups, saying that the majority of very poor women in the western capitalist, as well as developing, countries will never be able to afford the 'chance' to be helped by new technologies.

She is particularly disturbed about:

'neither the false promises and heavy burdens they impose on those who use them, nor the issue of unequal access to them, but their growing impact over the whole process of conception, pregnancy and childbirth and therefore on the concept of motherhood itself.'

(Foster 1995, p. 64)

Simple measures which might help to reduce the incidence and real pain of infertility in developed countries, she says, are left unimplemented:

'by an indifferent medical profession and societies in which the pursuit of profits takes precedence over the meeting of human needs.'

Her views make chilling reading when she concludes that we do not have to believe in male conspiracies to recognise that women may have already lost control over their reproductive lives. She is also critical of the health promotion strategies which purport to offer women real health choices and the opportunity to improve their health chances (and therefore those of their families). The 'pat' solutions they seem to offer, for example in suggestions about dietary change, fail to acknowledge cost and accessibility implications, and are also based on questionable findings:

'First, the type of dietary changes achieved by educating a free living group of subjects have proved to be relatively small. Second, the evidence that if achieved major dietary changes would save lives is also now seriously challenged.'

(Foster 1995, p. 145)

Investigations into high blood cholesterol and its links with heart disease, have, for example, been carried out almost exclusively on middle-aged men. The possibility of changing the fat content in one's diet to reduce the so-called 'bad' cholesterols could instead leave women open to the risk of osteoporosis (bone degeneration). Foster (1995) cites a Swedish study whereby the serum cholesterol of more than 10 000 middle-aged men was reduced over a 10 year period, only to find that the rate of deaths from coronary heart disease remained unchanged (see Oliver (1992) in Foster 1995, p. 146). The reader can detect a howl of heartfelt indignation in Foster's pleas for sanity to be restored:

'If eating a less fatty diet protects neither men nor women from premature death from cardiovascular disease why are women still being told by virtually all health experts that they should reduce their own and their families' consumption of saturated fats?'

(Foster 1995, p. 147)

Foster's thesis that the medicalisation of all women's problems is both disabling and disempowering is wide-ranging and convincing. Ann Oakley has similarly questioned the wisdom and morality of professional dominance over health care; and particularly maternity care, saying that in the contemporary industrialised world of medical science and allied disciplines, in claiming specialist jurisdiction over all aspects of reproduction, these disciplines have become the predominant source of social constructs of the culture of childbirth (Oakley 1993, p. 20). Oakley reminds us that even as far back as 1981 a World Health Organization (WHO) report was warning us that the three most common criticisms of health care expressed were that its benefits were distributed in an unequal way, that it has harmful effects (presumably as well as good?), and that modern health care is characterised by excessive technological intervention (WHO 1981).

Certainly women's sexuality has long been the 'target of religious and magical practices which have been mobilised to restrain women and to provide a surveillance of female reproductive capacity' (Turner 1995).

'Women's madness'

One of the problems associated with the biomedical model of 'mental illness' has been the observation that diagnostic categories are differentially distributed by gender, ethnicity and class, some of which may be put down to ethnocentrism or racist diagnostic practices, yet others to the conception that psychiatry as a branch of medicine:

'has been a male-dominated profession and has, thus, conveyed in its practices a male-orientated sense of normal psychological functioning.'

(see Samson 1995, p. 81 for an extensive discussion)

In a compelling account of the link between modern 'biological' psychiatry and women, the scholar Denise Russell suggests that from the nineteenth century onwards doctors have continued to dogmatically define women's madness in relation to a biological base for pragmatic reasons largely to do with power and influence:

'... firstly, to legitimise the entry of medicine into the new field of psychiatry, and, secondly, to further the moral guardianship role that medicine had taken on: medicine could act to curtail the protests of women about the constraints of the female role, as those protests were reconceptualized as mental symptoms of underlying physical pathology.'

(Russell 1995, p. 25)

Turner (1995) also observes that the flight into biology (my own expression) may have more to do with the criticisms made of established psychiatry, and the need for the profession to create a more acceptable role for itself within the context of the wider medical power base:

'One of the most important contributions of the "anti-psychiatry" writers has been to throw doubt on the validity of the concept of mental illness and the benevolence of psychiatric interventions.'

(Turner 1995, p. 78)

Obvious examples of the abuse of this kind of power could be the debates over women and 'tranquilliser' dependence on psychotropic drugs (see Foster 1995); another is the appropriation of the formerly widely contested diagnosis of 'premenstrual syndrome' now reclassified within the American Psychiatric Association's *Diagnostic and Statistical Manual of Mental Disorders* (Spitzer & Williams 1987) as 'late luteal dysphoric disorder' (see Russell 1995). It would seem, therefore, that in continuing to define a role for itself, biological psychiatry continues to depend on women for a clear sense of its identity!

From a late twentieth century perspective Russell examines the shifting trends in psychiatric diagnosis within 'biological psychiatry' and concludes overall that there might be convincing theoretical grounds on which to base a fresh start in trying to come to grips with human distress, particularly in relation to criminality:

'This is not a direction to kill the oppressor but rather to assist the oppressed. A theory of criminality could be developed where social change rather than individual correction would be taken as the best long-term strategy. The key would not be how to build better and bigger prisons to contain violence but how to develop a set of social relations such that violence is minimised.'

(Russell 1995, p. 162)

In allocating resources to health promotion the same value systems are seen to prevail. Because conventional health education is firmly rooted in a medical model of health placing the individual as the focus of implementation, the necessary changes in social structure to accommodate the aspirations of health care consumers is placed beyond reach. The continued use of clinically-orientated epidemiological studies to investigate the aetiology of disease has led to an undue tendency to seek explanations in terms of disease specific models:

'It is argued that to place primary emphasis on individual behaviour not only will be ineffective in reducing levels of disease, but also serves to draw attention away from those social, economic and environmental conditions which create vulnerability to disease and illness in the first place.'

(Research Unit in Health and Behavioural Change,
University of Edinburgh 1993, p. xvii)

Here the paradoxes of care and control can be detected clearly, as both patterns of dominance and control over suggested social 'deviance' from a government projected norm can be detected and exerted over the population within the rhetoric of health promotion. Turner describes this state of affairs as *bio-politics*, 'a stage in the secularisation of health and sickness in which the state has gradually replaced the Church as the central institution having control over life processes at the level of the individual and the household' (Turner 1995, p. 210). In trying to detect a comparative account of control over male fertility and subjugation the literature thins out considerably, with no convincing alternative critiques of human sexuality and health being offered as a counterweight to the notion of professional patriarchy over women.

Counterweights to medical power

When attempting to establish any counterweights to the power of doctors and society's medicalisation, some consideration has been given to the position of nurses within the medical hierarchy, with nursing being recognised as the paradoxical victim of a gender imbalance. Despite the fact that female nurses greatly outnumber their medical and managerial colleagues, they have not succeeded in challenging the status quo. As Larkin astutely observes, the state recognition of 'professions allied to medicine' has not effectively challenged the organising principles of the conventional medical division of labour, but rather accepted their embrace:

'Previous claims to an equality of professional status and scope of practice to doctors have been abandoned in exchange for state registration.'

(Larkin 1995, p. 53)

And as Witz has commented elsewhere, the challenge of the 'new' nursing as currently espoused in the UK has yet to be won.

Salvage believes that British nursing has entered a period of major change, promoted by a combination of pressures from within, difficulty in recruiting and retaining staff, significant educational reform and demands for higher status for women's work (Salvage 1992, p. 9). However, a close look at the reality of the organisation of nursing work shows both how it devalues the work of nursing and how it undermines and demeans the nurse herself (Davies 1995, p. 96). Witz, on the other hand, is sensitive to the likely effects of trends towards the decentralisation of health care finance and organisation, arguing that any global or collective vision of nursing in the future is likely to be rapidly displaced by local variations in the health division of labour.

Reflecting what has for some of us become personal experience, Witz believes that the development of nursing (far from being planned, as we've come to expect from the rhetoric of the nursing statutory bodies) will continue to develop pragmatically and in an ad hoc manner. The roles of doctors and health care managers in the new regime (particularly when you consider that former nurses now constitute a number of new generation managers) may well turn out to be critical as they seize opportunities to:

> 'shape the possibility and direction of change in nursing, as well as the nature of work and power relations between doctors and nurses.'
>
> (Witz in Gabe *et al.* 1994, p. 42)

As Walby *et al.* (1994) have noted, health work is atypical of other forms of contemporary industry because it is a *growth* industry. As demands for health care increase with the demographic shift in the age structure and as improvements in medical technology make more interventions possible, theories of employment, management and professionalisation will need to be revised to be consistent with these transformations (Walby *et al.* 1994, p. 3). There is also a timely reminder from Nicky James of Nottingham University, when she writes that nursing policy and social policy have so far failed to learn from each other (James 1992), although comparative policy discourse is gradually beginning to evolve in this area (for example Gough *et al.* 1994). May, for example, has stated categorically that the new nursing and the development of the new consumerism in health care do not sit comfortably with one another (May, C. 1995, p. 86). Bradshaw comments that the new nursing values of autonomy and empowerment, rejecting what is mistakenly and simplistically perceived to be the past nursing values of submission and obedience, have deconstructed the sense of continuity with the past, leading (it is argued) to a loss of authority in the present:

> 'These axioms have led to a new orthodoxy, which has brought fragmentation to the nursing profession as each nurse is taught to become a wholly autonomous practitioner; hence, the ward sister no longer inducts her charges into a tradition but rather takes on the role of a detached business manager.'
>
> (Bradshaw 1995, p. 304)

Somewhat ironically, the shift to budgetary control at ward level has diluted rather than distilled control over nursing functions: ward managers do not have the same authority to challenge budgets as more senior colleagues do, thus the shift of responsibility to ward managers is being accompanied by an increase in control by general managers (Alaszewski 1995, p. 65). Is this yet another example of the paradox of control?

The rise of consumerism

A further counterweight to medical power may be that of *consumer power*, the global response to many of the social and industrial changes taking place in a twentieth century dominated by the industrial might of the United States and the introduction of scientific management leading to a widespread culture of consumption (see Thompson 1994). The health policy analyst Rudolph Klein gives us some background as to the rise of consumerism in health care here in the UK:

'Social change brought about political change. If there was a new consumerism in the economic market place – epitomised by the rise of the supermarket chains – so also was there a new consumerism in the political market place. Politics became marked by diminishing partisanship and an increasing willingness to shop around among the parties.'

(Klein 1995, p. 134).

Brand loyalty could no longer be taken for granted and support, increasingly, came to depend on perceptions of performance (Klein 1995). The old ideologies bound up in working class votes for Labour and middle class votes for Conservatives no longer held good, as the boundaries separating the two had begun to blur in the smelting of individualist aspirations to wealth of the Thatcher era, and in *postmodern* trends to abandon the old 'grand' ideologies of socialism and capitalism in favour of new discourses in economics, gender, class and social influence (see George & Wilding 1994). Some have even gone so far as to talk about the *post-welfare state* (personal communication, 1995).

Klein observes a further paradox in health care consumerism, in that the transformation of patient to consumer is a response to top-down policies, rather than to bottom-up demands. Overall he concludes that radical change, in whatever direction to realign health, will always be perceived publicly as disruptive. The uncertainties and upheavals created by the reforms of the NHS (as in life as a whole) have generated, in turn, a demand for stability and predictability. It therefore follows, in Klein's view, that the search for a new equilibrium will constrain the ability of *any* government (his italics) to adopt radical policies of change. Government needs to develop the flexibility to adapt to an uncertain future:

'The NHS is therefore likely to remain a self-inventing institution, responding incrementally both to the evolving and unpredictable pattern of health care delivery and to the ideological biases of whichever party happens to be in power.'

(Klein 1995, p. 253)

Science, caring and the consumer

It is claimed that our awe of science and technology has had consequences for the power of professionals and that its consequences have negatively influenced the value and definition of 'caring' within health work (Hawthorne & Yurkovich 1995). Patient satisfaction studies which are purported to build on the concept of consumer sovereignty (and are therefore perceived as a product of the orientation to consumerism) are methodologically speaking complex, and open to multiple interpretations (see Batchelor *et al.* 1994). Any discussion of the impact of new technologies on individuals and their families is not made explicit in qualitative and quantitative analyses of study outcomes, other than to elucidate degrees of technical success. Far-reaching claims are made for the perceived benefits of technological advancement, and it is arguably important to place these developments within a human framework.

The Paradox of Technological Arrogance

Gloomy predictions of the outcomes of our technological arrogance, the refutation of the presumption that science knows what is best for us, ought to be resisted according to Arthur Caplan, director of the Center for Bioethics at the University of Pennsylvania Medical Center, and founding President of the American Association of Bioethics. Predicted financial ruin and despair, based on intractable problems of demographics and limited money, negate the many benefits which could potentially accrue to us if we embraced the dynamic possibilities science offers.

Caplan asks vital, life-defining questions. Current preoccupations with gene therapy bring us face to face with questions about the malleability and perfectibility of our species:

'Is the emerging revolution in medical technology one that will leave us so befuddled about who we are that we will one day look back longingly for simpler times when children died of illnesses such as Tay-Sachs disease, sickle cell anaemia and cystic fibrosis, and adults were ravaged by cancer, diabetes and heart disease?'

(Caplan 1995, p. 111)

Why should changing our 'biological blueprints' in pursuit of longer, healthier lives pose any more of a threat than our own ability to improve human health by taking impurities out of the water supply, Caplan asks. As he says, we have gradually been altering our gene pool over thousands of years through the effects of wars, selective mating, improved diet and the evolution of scientific medicine. He agrees, however, that we need to tread carefully in seeing that genetic engineering is not misused:

'we must guard diligently against misuse of the ability to design our descendants with careful regulation, legislation and societal consensus.'

(Caplan 1995, p. 111)

He argues that if being human means using intelligence to improve the quality of our lives, then there is little basis for ethical ambivalence about eliminating genetic scourges, much as we have done in the past with infectious diseases such as polio and smallpox.

It would seem to the non-scientist, however, that the essential paradox here lies in our aspirations to human perfectibility: like the earlier paradox of holism in relation to alternative health movements, if human beings were intended to be perfect, how is it that our intelligence has taken us this long to arrive at a possible solution? In terms of human experience, it is our frailties and individual differences which make us unique. It is hard to comprehend a world where bodily perfection is the norm. And anyway, are we to assume that the non-diseased body would be spiritually benevolent and intact? Also, if it is the ultimate paradox, the fear of death itself, which motives us to live, will we no longer have a death to fear? If we have no bodily decay, will we have to engineer our own deaths to criteria agreed legislatively and societally in response to the changes proposed?

These are questions which are neither hypothetical, far-fetched nor aesthetic in character, but practical, in view of the megatrends affecting the sophisticated advances in medical technology. In less then a century we have already come to offer life support in a manner which would have seemed other-worldly to our great grandparents; for example in open heart surgery and renal dialysis. As if to reassure us, Caplan concludes with the following:

'If we can make that future affordable, if we can enhance the quality of our lives while controlling population growth, and if we can accept the idea that it is neither arrogant nor foolhardy to modify our biological constitution in the hope of preventing disorder and disease, medical technology could very well make the future better'

(Caplan 1995, p. 111)

Given that this commentary appeared in the 150th anniversary issue of the prestigious journal *Scientific American,* one couldn't really expect any radical alternative vision of science. To the non-scientist, however, Caplan's final statement includes a great many 'ifs'.

The Paradox of Human Communication

The distinguished Australian surgeon, Miles Little (1995) has an alternative mission, however, for the development of a *humane medicine,* even though he recognises that the reductionist science of a bio-mechanical model of human disease is insufficient for the task. Without an ethical base, he believes that reductionist science can indeed become corrupt. Better communication is necessary between doctors and their patients if patients are to be treated humanely.

Skills of empathy are required. Barriers to human communication are formed between doctor and patient by a media hostile to, and unappreciative of, the problems confronting the medical establishment. Public expectations are fuelled by the media, leading to a confusion of wants and needs:

'Once formed, expectations are difficult to change, particularly when it is necessary to lower them. A culture of science and materialism creates expectations that the power of science can solve any problem.'

(Little 1995, p. 176)

Little concedes that medicine unwittingly encourages these expectations by emphasising science over human understanding:

'The empirical, positivist element in medicine has overwhelmed the humane, devaluing discourse and rendering language less important than objective measurements and structural appearances. The reward and granting systems within medicine continue to signal that positivism is good, and that value-laden endeavour is worthy but ultimately suspect. The human genome project will attract more support than any research and practice in palliative care.'

(Little 1995, p. 176)

What he describes as the 'market element' in medicine is also ethically problematic, and the rhetoric of the marketplace may also interfere with the language of human communication. On a broader plane, the 'rhetoric of efficiency' has been blamed elsewhere for driving an ideological wedge between health service providers and their 'consumers', leading to a perceived erosion in the human service 'capital' which is said to exist within the psyche of health workers (see Wilkinson 1995).

The development of humane communication

Attempts to develop collaborative and interprofessional working in health care has met with varying degrees of success, although any attempts to redraw the cultural boundaries between different occupational groups may themselves be seen as a drain on the morale and energy resources of an already depressed workforce. As Professor Alan Beattie has observed in his prospective 'new republic of health':

> 'the very possibility of making a transition from traditional tribal boundaries in health to a different division of labour, will itself depend on action also at "macro" level. If the traditional classes and castes of the health professions are to be replaced by new health cadres and health teams, a great deal of energy and imagination will need to go into the design of new managerial systems to support them.'

> (Beattie 1995, p. 21)

Whether new managerial systems will rise to this challenge is open to conjecture. Managerial support for organisational change tends to support the status quo in terms of organisational hierarchy, with culture change still being viewed as an imposition rather than a shared response to new cultural forces (see Pettigrew *et al.* (1992) for a detailed review of NHS change strategies). The everyday practical dilemmas faced by health workers in a cost-constrained environment have led to the introduction of more explicit policies of 'whistle-blowing' as regards poor performance or unethical practices against the interests of the service or its consumers; in effect, a successful attempt to depoliticise structural defects in the health care system by apportioning blame to individuals.

Certainly my own experience, and the anecdotal reports of my 'significant others', would suggest that tribalism also extends to those in the service who are perceived as loyal to managerial rather than 'health professional' objectives, so that the differentiation and delineation of specific roles in health care come to represent different claims to the moral high ground in arguments and debates about power relationships (at the macro level), or in decision making about resources at the 'micro' level. Hence it is possible for nurses and doctors to argue that they have the patient's best interests at heart, while managers are relegated to a (perceived) lesser sub-territory, that of the general state of the budget and financial analysis. Disputes arising from organisational and managerial priority-taking no doubt account for a disproportionate amount of time in multidisciplinary meetings, for example. Setting one section of the workforce against another (or even to induce internal division, for example, within nursing) is an effective divide and rule strategy for managers wishing to gain the controlling hand of deliberations. Reported low morale and dispiritedness in nursing is exemplified in the continuing need for supportive role models and a recognition that nursing is, above all, a human activity (Morton-Cooper & Palmer 1993). Models of *clinical supervision*, which are ostensibly designed to empower nursing, therefore have the same effect as any other subversively 'controlling' strategy – yet another example of paradox – in that nurses who make claims to be autonomous have their autonomy strictly relegated to a borrowed and rapidly diminishing power base within the medical hierarchy (Morton-Cooper 1995).

Communication and managerial role

Human communication is by nature hazardous. The psychosocial forces which underpin our reactions to situations – outward bodily gestures, internalised feelings – again hark back to those fragile (and contested) connections between our perceptions of mind and body. A critical examination of everyday communication between colleagues in the form of rigorous discourse methodology is not always practical or helpful. Where formal studies have been conducted health care professionals have been taken to task for their failure to communicate as empathetically and straightforwardly as we might imagine. Defensive strategies may be employed, particularly when emotive or deeply personal issues are discussed, and wittingly or otherwise communication is compromised by such tactics as withholding information, refusing to evaluate or comment on the performance of a colleague, and discrediting patients by negating the individual's claims to discomfort or illness through dismissive or over-assertive language (see Nichols (1984) for a discussion on the clinical psychologist's perspective on 'informational care'). Effective communication between colleagues, or between carers and their clients, are interpreted via sensory processes which may be more 'controllable' than we realise.

The qualities of the voice are an important mediator of communication and are seen as strong determinants of effectiveness, for example, concerning resonance, rhythm, speed, pitch, voice inflection and clarity (see Hunsaker & Alessandra, cited in Leddy & Pepper 1992, p. 296). Accompanying motor movements, or *kinesics*, can also be significant from a common-sense perspective, but it is useful to remember that body movements are non-verbal communications which developed in a particular psychosocial and cultural setting which may vary according to gender, socio-economic status, age and ethic background (Leddy & Pepper 1992, p. 296). In health care, communication is often related to some form of crisis, either of the emotional transition variety (such as early bereavement, loss, anticipatory grieving, pain, anxiety) or in the longer term adjustments to a life change. Whether the crisis is perceived as temporary or permanent, different strategies for people management or direct care-giving are necessary to manage this crisis effectively. The dawn of psychological contracting as discussed earlier in this book, is one obvious area for the development of communication skills which are able to address the adaptation and resolution phases of crisis management. For managers themselves, this may include some form of *conflict identification* and *resolution*.

Bad things can happen to good managers, as Marelli points out (Marelli 1993, p. 254):

- You may be promoted when your friend is not.
- You may feel discomfort in an unfamiliar environment.
- You may experience times of stress, conflict and 'high anxiety'.
- You may be disheartened when your own managers fail to keep their promises.
- You may not feel your manager is competent.
- Your managerial training or preparation may be inadequate.
- You may inherit problems from previous managers.
- Your manager may negatively evaluate your performance.
- You may not get the recognition you deserve.

Conflict management

On a more theoretical note, it may be useful to develop sensory antennae for recognising the difference between constructive and destructive conflicts. This isn't necessarily easy as many conflicts remain destructive because people cannot pull together the communication skills necessary for constructive problem-solving (Donohue & Kolt 1992). Leadership competence is of note here, as one of the most powerful ways people deal with potential embarrassment is to create *organisational defensive routines* (Argyris 1992, p. 84). These routines can impact on the goodwill involved in the psychological contract between employers and their staff. Argyris defines the organisational defensive routine as:

'any action or policy that prevents human beings from experiencing negative surprises, embarrassment, or threat, and simultaneously prevents the organisation from reducing or eliminating the cause of the surprises, embarrassment or threat. Organisational defensive routines are anti-learning and overprotective.'

(Argyris 1992, p. 84)

Conflicts which appear at the time to be destructive may later reveal themselves as constructive and vice versa (Donohue & Kolt 1992). In setting down some evaluative criteria for conflict management and recognition, Donohue and Kolt describe *constructive conflicts* as interest centred, openly manifest, capable of bolstering interdependence (i.e. 'binding together'), focused on flexible means for solving the dispute.

Destructive conflicts on the other hand may be needs centred, focused on personalities and not behaviours, involved in power preservation and 'face-saving', aimed at compromising interdependence (and therefore likely to destroy trust and incite revenge). These conflicts involve the use of attacking and defending comments, leading to escalation of conflict which may then lend themselves to at best avoidance, and at worst, violence. These authors say that there are three important issues at stake here which need to be worked through in order to develop workable interpersonal relationships, they are *control, trust* and *intimacy*. Language and power strategies are involved in any attempt to 'power balance', to negotiate effectively and to survive any conflict with dignity and 'face' (Donohue & Kolt 1992)

Business ethics and health care management

Professional service organisations are having to change the way they are managed in order to produce an ethical environment which will allow managers and staff to power balance with a degree of integrity in the face of more pragmatic demands, and ethicality is beginning to be viewed as an important characteristic of the healthy post-modern organisation (see Newell 1995). Successful negotiation as a manager may be affected by different conceptions of what a manager is or does; for example, whether management is by 'facilitation' or alternatively by 'constraint'. It is clear that the strategic issue of professionalising the management function in health care was a major concern of the British NHS in the 1980s and that the territorial boundaries laid then may still be shifting (Dawson 1994).

Communication as organisational problem-solving

Organisational culture is a subject which until recently has failed to capture the serious attention of researchers (Bate 1992). On the subject of 'culture' itself, Bate makes the common-sense observation that culture is predominantly *implicit* (his italics) in people's minds; it is not something that is 'out there' with a separate existence of its own; neither is it directly observable. Bate's own research into three organisations attempted to identify those aspects of each culture which had a strong impact on organisational problem-solving. He reports that, to a greater or lesser extent, the following characteristics were present:

- unemotionality
- depersonalisation
- subordination
- conservatism
- isolationism
- antipathy.

'Unemotionality' was reflected in the apparent superficiality of work relationships. In the case of managers, sharing feelings and emotions was construed as a sign of being unprofessional, as a weakness or inefficiency. As Bate observed:

'People's lack of ability to engage in meaningful interaction was painfully obvious in meetings that did take place; "We all want to discuss common problems but when we actually get there most of us are fairly mute" (junior manager). and "Our meetings? In a word – weak. Lukewarm affairs" (shop steward). "People never really open up about their concerns. It means that our meetings are pretty dry affairs ... I suppose we are all fairly reluctant to bring our dirty washing into the open" (personnel officer).'

(Bate 1992, p. 221)

The irony here is that the link between poor communication and work-related causes of stress are well documented. Internal conflicts, role ambiguity, role overload and (conversely) underload are all recognised contributors to job stress, with social support being a significant factor in the reduction of stress experienced in the 'healthy organisation' (Newell 1995). The perception that honest, open communication is 'dirty washing' to be worked through privately is presumably an important demotivator in coming to terms with work place problems. The relationship between motivation and emotion is nevertheless gaining new ground as a legitimate subject for study. For example, it is argued that cultural rules about appropriate conduct guide the behaviour of the people around us and directly constrain or facilitate certain forms of emotion in social life (Parkinson 1995).

Emotions and roles are intertwined in complex ways. As Parkinson says, different societies have different conventions about the appropriateness of different emotions. To have their intended effects,

> 'our actions must be meaningful to other people and must therefore conform to shared conventions of significance.'
>
> (Parkinson 1995, p. 203)

Parkinson notes that we cannot start from scratch and invent completely new ways of communicating or influencing one another. Existing social frameworks will always mediate our communications:

> 'Most of social life (as well as the architectural arrangements that support it) is set up so that you are in contact only with people that it is necessary or appropriate (from the point of view of the surrounding organization or culture) to communicate with, and this places obvious limits on the range of emotions and emotional objects that are available.'
>
> (Parkinson 1995, p. 204)

One classic example of this from the patient's perspective is the spectacle which revolves around the consultant physician or surgeon's 'ward round'. Patients have been prepared for this great visit by nurses scurrying about, tidying up and signalling to patients that the big moment is about to arrive:

> 'Sister will raise her eyebrow or nod in approval at the patient's performance in maintaining the drama. The patient who tries to call the Consultant back; who tries to ignore the rules, will be "shushed" and told by the sister "I'll come back and talk to you later". There is to be no denting of the performance; no possibility that the measured progression of the Consultant is to be interrupted. The occasional "common touch" of the Consultant will be demonstrated when he lifts the book on your locker and makes a little comment on it before moving on to the next performer-cum-audience.'
>
> (Mackay 1993, p. 112)

Mackay has a serious point. The need for a performance by which the status of medicine is always maintained is real. Patients take innocent comments and read all manner of sinister inferences into them. They look for certainties where none can be promised. Faith in treatments must be protected and maintained by this elaborate dramatic presentation. The consent of the patient is, after all, critical. As Mackay illustrates, without the co-operation of the patient, anarchy would reign:

> 'Few patients yell at the Consultant; few patients swear at a doctor, yet in their ordinary life every sentence may contain an expletive. As

children we learn those doctor–patient games and by the time we are grown-ups we have learned them by heart.'

(Mackay 1993, p. 112)

Parkinson's book *Ideas and Realities of Emotion* contains a stimulating and challenging view of the institutional factors affecting emotional performance in service industries, including concepts of 'emotional alienation' which could make insightful and revelatory reading for managers in health care (Parkinson 1995). For a more general discussion on the subject of emotions at work see Rafaeli and Sutton (1995). An overview of the psychology literature on emotion and motivation is discussed in a short book by Parkinson & Colman (1995), and a detailed analysis of the concept of 'emotional contagion' within human communication (the medical model extends even to this!) is contained within a more detailed text by Hatfield *et al.* (1994).

Taking all of these points into consideration, it would appear that the *paradox of human communication* lies in our apparent inability to communicate instinctively. Whether we are attempting to communicate formally or informally, at whatever level of abstraction or certainty, we do need to constantly re-evaluate the practices and assumptions which underpin or underlie practice. The problems arising from this have perplexed philosophers and political commentators for millennia; but what is clear is that any intelligible theory of organisational life must be coherent within prevailing conceptions of the human being (Gergen 1992, p. 208). Our failure to adapt to, and take account of, the complexities of human communication in the everyday conduct of our affairs is to effectively devalue the currency of communication which allows us to participate in (as well as 'manage') our living and working relationships.

The dawn of the 'new age' manager?

Although sensitivity as a quality might seem to be at odds with our perception of an aggressive 'lean, mean' business ethos, there is a growing concern with business leaders to respond appropriately to the express needs of clients (clients could equally well include employees). Hickman and Silva take this view of the situation in their text on building excellence in business life:

'All people want their needs and expectations fulfilled by the organisations they choose to work for. Otherwise, they bide their time or resign. In either case, morale plunges and productivity declines. Turnover in personnel and deteriorating productivity are sure signs of organisational *in*sensitivity.'

(Hickman & Silva 1984, p. 129)

Supportive leadership in health care

Supportive behaviours help build and maintain effective interpersonal relationships. A manager who is considerate and friendly towards people is more likely to win their friendship and loyalty (Yukl 1994). Whether or not you agree with this view, it is likely that you have an opinion of the value or otherwise of your own support networks as a manager.

One of the key difficulties identified in defining business leadership is that representations of leadership tend to assume that leadership itself is a quality invested in individuals rather than groups. Andrew Wall (1989) has written that a thorough understanding of the ethical implications of health managers' work should enhance their standing and reputation. He declares that regardless of apparent pressures on the system, the goal of managers in health care is to see that the care and treatment of patients respects the individual and the common goals of the organisation at the same time. He acknowledges that the choices and decisions facing managers may be complex, and well beyond the simple checklist to perform. Good ethical behaviour, if I interpret him correctly, is 'exemplified by staff doing their best whatever the circumstances' (Wall 1989, p. 92). The law, for example, cannot be relied upon to salvage a solution:

'The law and ethics are by no means synonymous. The statute book endeavours to be absolute and unambiguous, but many ethical dilemmas depend for their resolution upon the evaluation of interrelated factors. For most people working in the health service, the law is invoked more to placate anxiety than for any other reason; it suggests certainty in an uncertain and potentially dangerous environment. In such a climate managers need to be able to hold on to ethical principles in order to protect the interests of patients and staff even when the law appears not to.'

(Wall 1989, p. 93)

It could also be argued that it is possible to develop a supportive managerial strategy based on leadership which, if taken to its logical conclusion, will permeate the work culture at various levels. Yukl reports that a meta-analysis of results from a large number of studies on supportive behaviours by managers demonstrated that: 'subordinates of supportive leaders are usually more satisfied with their leaders and their jobs' (see Fisher & Edwards 1988 cited in Yukl 1994, p. 119). The management theorist Tony Watson interviewed managers and asked them questions such as 'What is the most important thing in life to you?' and 'Can you identify any personal values or beliefs that you think are relevant to the way you work?' The answers can be revealing, or can result in the 'standard respectable answer' in Watson's experience (Watson 1994, p. 75).

From these elementary questions, it may still be possible to elicit the strength and nature of morale among managers, and identify opportunities to develop more sensitive behaviours and management structures.

For those who aspire to recognition as *transformational leaders*, Yukl discusses a study which found such leaders had the following attributes:

- They saw themselves as change agents.
- They were prudent risk-takers.
- They believed in people and were sensitive to their needs.
- They were able to articulate a set of core values which guided their behaviour.
- They were flexible and open to learning from experience.
- They had cognitive skills and believed in disciplined thinking and the need for careful analysis of problems.
- They were visionaries who trusted their own intuition.

(See Yukl 1994, p. 363 for a comprehensive discussion.) This last attribute, which alights on the relative powers of intuition is an enlightening one, particularly given its possible relationship with instinctive communication as discussed earlier in this section.

Given that health reform can lead to significant cultural change within the health services (Strike 1995), the after-effects of those changes and their consequent 'fall-out' are likely to tax the managers' capacity for effective communication, personally and professionally, for some time to come. The transformations which evolve will be far-reaching, requiring a 'good-enough' resolution to the paradox of human communication in the interests of working relationships (productivity?) as well as the greater good of society as the consumer and arbiter of health care as a whole.

The Paradox of Public 'Charterism'

The search for excellence in health care

The pursuit of excellence in health care appears to be only one aspect of a 'growing recognition that the delivery of welfare involves much more than value for money; and what Gunn has described as the fourth "E" to add to Economy, Efficiency and Effectiveness, *Excellence*' (Gunn, cited in Butcher 1995).

Butcher himself traces the concern with excellence to the influential

American writers Tom Peters and Robert Waterman, authors of the best-selling book *In Search of Excellence* (1982) which sets out the basic principles of their approach to business excellence. One of these principles was a need to be close to the customer. 'Excellent' companies are those dominated by an organisational culture which focuses on customer's preferences and caters to them:

> 'Customers were not regarded as a nuisance or ignored, but were regularly listened to, with companies often getting some of their best ideas from them. "Excellent" companies had what amounted to an "obsession" with customer service.'
>
> (Butcher 1995, p. 138)

When the American economist Alain Einthoven conducted his influential review of the British NHS in 1985, he concluded that there were several fundamental obstacles to development, which Renade (1994, p. 57) has described as:

- poor matching of funding to workload
- inappropriate incentives and mixed rewards for managers and clinicians
- lack of responsiveness to consumers
- few incentives to innovate or to remain cost-conscious and cost-efficient.

Proposed corrective reforms for these anomalies were laid out in the white paper *Working for Patients* issued by the Department of Health (DoH) in January 1989. John Butler, professor of health studies at the University of Kent has observed that the white paper was rather better at describing the symptoms of perceived maladies in the NHS than in making any constructive diagnosis:

> 'Different causes may require different remedies; yet the white paper was innocent of any analysis of why the excesses had arisen, why they had failed to respond adequately to previous ameliorative attempts, or why the new treatment would do the trick where others had failed.'
>
> (Butler 1992, p. 48)

An evaluation of the recent changes initiated by the Conservative government's NHS and Community Care Act 1990 by Gladstone and Goldsmith (1995) describes the changes brought about as a considerable contrast to the original vision of the market as expressed in the first white paper. Attempts to soften the language of the market in order to bolster support for the reforms ultimately led to changes in the terminology used. New terms were devised to describe new elements in the reform process, which the authors say were never envisaged either by think-tanks or the government; changes which in Gladstone and Goldsmith's view ultimately compounded the problems of reform.

Because no independent non-governmental system was established to monitor or evaluate the reforms, the production of any kind of reliable balance sheet as to their successes is problematic, particularly when set alongside the new contract for GPs, the *Health of the Nation* targets and the *Patient's Charter* initiative (Gladstone & Goldsmith 1995, p. 80). The authors' overall conclusion is that there are three tensions which are either a result of or a reflection on pre-existing conditions and turbulence within the service. The first is the need to prioritise effectively. The second concerns the prospects for resolution of the tensions between the 'free market' and central government regulation; and the third concerns the tension between medical professionals, managers and consumers.

The extent to which the consumer voice holds up in all of this has also been well criticised. The journalist Annabelle May has no doubts about the relative successes of charter initiatives in health care:

'Communication between the public and the NHS has come to resemble Monty Python's semaphore version of Wuthering Heights where Cathy and Heathcliff attempt to convey their passion by frantically signalling to each other from separate mountain peaks. But judging by the avalanche of consumer-related proposals emerging, concern is mounting that the rhetoric of patient choice, charters and community involvement has raised expectations which the system has so far failed to fulfil.'

(May, A. 1995)

The proverbial jury would therefore currently appear to be out on determining the best way to assess consumer opinion of health reforms (although a ministerial review is apparently under way at the time of writing). In principle, at least, it is worth considering the aims behind the concept of public 'charterism' and what it appears to signify to partakers and providers of health care here in the UK and perhaps to onlookers in other health care economies.

The advent of public 'charterism'

There can be no doubt that models of service evaluation, quality assurance, audit and related issues are currently high on a number of agendas (Nolan & Grant 1993). The *Patient's Charter* (DoH 1991, 1995) is but one of a number of social services charters stemming from the government's *Citizen's Charter Initiative* (HMSO 1991) which was officially launched in a white paper in July 1991. The stated purpose of the initiative was to improve the quality of public services and to make them more responsive to their users (see Butcher (1995) for a contextual review).

Butcher explains that the Citizen's Charter had four main themes: to improve the quality of public services; to provide choice, wherever possible, between competing providers; to inform citizens as to what service standards are and how to act where they deem service to be unacceptable; and, lastly, to give full value for money within a tax bill that the nation could afford (Butcher 1995, p. 149).

Alongside this more specific models of service evaluation were considered a vital element of service delivery, although 'the rhetoric is more difficult to translate into reality' (Nolan & Grant 1993). Measurement is at best a precarious business, as the Radical Statistics Health Group (RSHG) discovered when it attempted to analyse the accuracy of the government's official 'indicators of success' (RSHG 1995, p. 1045). Instead, they concluded that there is a real danger that in trying to achieve targets linked to a relatively narrow set of indicators, staff's attention may be distracted from other issues, notably the quality, effectiveness and appropriateness of the clinical care provided (RSHG 1995, p. 1048).

Not only is there evidence to suggest that mental illness is rising in health service staff as a result of conflicting pressures and demands, in a system which is accused of 'abandoning caring for the ethos of the balance sheet', (Bird 1995, p. 18) a report from the DoH which encourages doctors to 'whistle-blow' on incompetent colleagues creates the potential for internal division and distrust among health care colleagues when they are attempting to work collaboratively (DoH 1995). Internal strife and mutual suspicion, irrespective of the wider professional priority to put the interests of patients first, is hardly likely to inspire the transformational models of leadership and cohesive teamwork necessary to high quality care.

Managing the quality of a service therefore depends very much on your personal perspective. Whose 'standards' (in the broadest sense of the word) are we to measure care by? All standards are, by definition, relative to the stated aim of care. As Baddeley has written in an overview of Patient's Charter ethics from a doctor's perspective, there is a strong possibility that the 'Charter Rights' laid out for patients may sow the seed of confusion between what constitutes different standards and measures of quality. He senses a danger in that the general public may come to equate measurable but largely irrelevant statistics – such as waiting times – with the relatively unquantifiable, but in his view much more important, standard of quality of care (Baddeley 1995, p. 50). He also wonders whether NHS Trusts may direct resources into areas in which administrators know they can achieve measurable standards (e.g.

orthopaedic surgery) and away from areas in which outcome is much more difficult to quantify.

From the point of view of senior health care managers (in both private and public sectors of care), the publication of the Patient's Charter might have enabled them to question clinicians and insist on adherence to pre-ordained standards (Wall 1995). The limitations of the Charter soon became clear, however, as Wall explains, when managers became concerned that standards laid down in the Charter could be used as the basis for subsequent league tables of performance, making invidious comparisons between one part of the NHS and another. Valuable though comparisons may be as an indicator for further analysis

'they are also potentially dangerous if used naively, causing unfair and damaging opinions to be passed on to those who may be working under particular difficulties.'

(Wall 1995, p. 77)

He questions whether the Charter is being used instrumentally to bring about change and to 'call to heel' the managers and clinicians within the NHS. Wall concludes that those who were sceptical of the government's motives probably had a right to be so, even if it was not unreasonable of the government to 'overcome entrenched attitudes in a public service not renowned for its ability to change practices' (Wall 1995, p. 78). Calling for a more detailed analysis of the ethics of charterism, he is, on balance, optimistic about the future:

'The Charter can provide a check, a balance, a stimulus and a reminder that, ethically, the NHS stands as being a brave attempt to maximise the benefits to the whole of society, while honouring obligations to each particular patient. Managers have their place in endeavouring to resolve this seeming paradox.'

(Wall 1995, p. 103)

The game of wizards and gatekeepers

Whether or not you share this optimism, it is hard to negate any sincere attempts (however cosmetic or superficial you might suppose them to be) to chart the wishes of the recipients of a service; particularly one which touches everyone to some degree or other across their lifespan. In a humorous stab at the 'system' to emerge from recent national health reform here in the UK, Herd *et al.* (1995) devised an elaborate tale of modern allegory, in an issue of the *British Medical Journal.* Imaginatively entitled *The Wizard and the Gatekeeper: of Castles and Contracts,* it reads:

'The wizards and the gatekeepers were unhappy ... the poorly people's charter was resulting in unrealistic expectations... There were
still lots of poorly people who couldn't be cured, and some of the
magic potions were a bit unpredictable, with no-one knowing how
they actually worked. Some of the new ones were very expensive. The
wizards started asking if the King and his chancellor wanted these new
spells, and if so, how they were to be paid for. "More efficiency!"
howled the minister; "No more money!" chanted the chancellor; "The
wizards and the gatekeepers must compete for poorly people!" roared
the King.

(Herd *et al.* 1995, p. 1042)

While we can (and must!) laugh about the paradoxes evident in
modern health care, if only to preserve what remains of our collective
sanity, the serious point still remains that some structural commitment
needs to be made to tackle the widespread disillusionment and cynicism
which threatens our continued assault on the problems. Alan Cribb
(1995) has asked the critical question:

'Will the introduction of market values, competition, and incentives
into the UK health service undermine the traditional values of the
service, and the nature of care?'

He considers that the traditional values of health care will be defended
by professional integrity, and by professional commitment to the practices of care. But will all these paradoxes *ever* be resolved? Cribb
believes that the key question concerns not whether the values intrinsic
to care will be maintained alongside professional and institutional
rewards. He tells us that there is no health system which does not
depend upon these things co-existing. Rather, the key question is how
best they can be maintained, requiring consideration of both moral
psychology and sociology; a position reinforced, I hope, by our detailed
consideration of modern social and moral paradox:

'Can it be left to the virtues of clear-headed individuals to insulate the
intrinsic from the instrumental values? More realistically, we should
ask whether we can create structures and cultures which act as
insulators, and which help individual professionals to strike a balance
between private and public interests, and between health gain and
care.'

(Cribb 1995, p. 181)

Or, as Alvin Toffler (1977) has foretold, diagnosis precedes cure. We
cannot begin to help ourselves until we become sensitively conscious of
the problem. It is only by making imaginative use of change to *channel*

change that we can not only spare ourselves the trauma of future shock, but reach out and humanise our distant tomorrows.

References

Alaszewski, A. (1995) Restructuring health and welfare professions in the United Kingdom: the impact of internal markets on the medical, nursing and social work professions. In: *Health Professions and the State in Europe*, (eds T. Johnson, G. Larkin & M. Saks). Routledge, London.

Argyris, C. (1992) A leadership dilemma: skilled incompetence. In: *Human Resources Strategies*, (ed. G. Salaman). Sage/Open University, London.

Baddeley, P. (1995) A doctor's view. In: *Ethics – the Patient's Charter*, (ed V. Tschudin). Scutari Press, London.

Barker, J.R.V. (1955) *The Brontes*. Phoenix Giants, London.

Batchelor, C., Owens D.J., Read, M. & Bloor, M. (1994) Patient satisfaction studies: methodology, management and consumer evaluation. *International Journal of Health Care Quality Assurance*, **7**(7), 22–30.

Bate, P. (1992) The impact of organizational culture on approaches to organizational problem-solving. In: *Human Resources Strategies*, (ed. G. Salaman). Sage/Open University, London.

Beattie, A. (1995) War and peace among the health tribes. In: *Interprofessional Relations in Health Care*, (eds K. Soothill, L. Mackay & C. Webb). Edward Arnold, London.

Beveridge, W. (1942) *Social Insurance and Allied Services; Report by Sir William Beveridge*. Cmnd 6404. HMSO, London.

Bird, J. (1995) Sick nurses or a sick NHS? *Nursing Standard*, **9**(49), 18–19.

Bradshaw, A. (1995) Nursing and medicine: co-operation or conflict? In: Has nursing lost its way? (J.A. Short) *British Medical Journal*, **311**, 303–308.

Butcher, T. (1995) *Delivering Welfare: the Governance of the Social Services in the 1990s*. Open University Press, Buckingham.

Butler, J. (1992) *Patients, Policies and Politics: Before and After* Working for Patients. Open University Press, Buckingham.

Caplan, A. (1995) An improved future? Medical advances challenging thinking on living, dying and being human. *Scientific American*, **273**(3), 110–11.

Christie, B. (1995a) Tried, not tested. *The Scotsman* 1 November.

Christie, B. (1995b) Doctors' fears over brain disease in two teenagers. *The Scotsman*, 27 October.

Clayre, A. (ed.) (1977) *Nature and Industrialization*. Oxford University Press in association with Open University Press, Oxford.

Coward, R. (1989) *The Whole Truth: the Myth of Alternative Health*. Faber & Faber, London.

Cribb, A. (1995) A turn for the better? Philosophical issues in evaluating health care reforms. In: *Reforming Health Care: The Philosophy and Practice of International Health Reform*, (ed. D. Seedhouse). John Wiley & Sons, Chichester.

Davies, C. (1995) *Gender and the Professional Predicament in Nursing*. Open University Press, Buckingham.

Dawson, S. (1994) Changes in the distance: professionals reappraise the meaning of management. *Journal of General Management*, **2**(1), 1–21.

DoH (1991) *The Patient's Charter*. HMSO, London.

DoH (1995) *The Patient's Charter*. HMSO, London.

DoH (1995) *Monitoring Medical Excellence*. HMSO, London.

Donohue, W.A. & Kolt, R. (1992) *Managing Interpersonal Conflict*. Sage, California.

Drife, J. & Johnston, I. (1995) Handling the conflicting cultures in the NHS. *British Medical Journal*, **310**, 1054–6.

Feldman, M.D. & Ford, C.V. (1994) *Patient or Pretender: Inside the Strange World of Factitious Disorders*. John Wiley & Sons, New York.

Fisher, B.M. & Edwards, J.E. (1988) *Consideration and initiating structure and their relationships with leader effectiveness: a meta-analysis. Proceedings of the Academy of Management*, August, 201–205.

Foster, P. (1995) *Women & the Health Care Industry: an Unhealthy Relationship?* Open University Press, Buckingham.

Gabe, J., Kelleher, D. & Williams, G. (1994) *Challenging Medicine*. Routledge, London.

George, V. & Wilding, P. (1994) *Welfare and Ideology*. Harvester Wheatsheaf, Hemel Hempstead.

Gergen, K.J. (1992) Organization theory in the postmodern era. In: *Rethinking Organization: New Directions in Organization Theory and Analysis* (eds M. Reed & M. Holroyd). Sage, London.

Gladstone, D. & Goldsmith M. (1995) Health care reform in the UK: working for patients? In: *Reforming Health Care: The Philosophy and Practice of Health Reform*, (ed. D. Seedhouse). John Wiley & Sons, Chichester.

Gough, P., Maslin-Prothero, S. & Masterson, A. (1994) *Nursing and Social Policy: Care in Context*. Butterworth-Heinemann, Oxford.

Granshaw, L. (1992) The rise of the modern hospital in Britain. In: *Medicine in Society: Historical Essays* (ed. A. Wear). Cambridge University Press, Cambridge.

Handy, C. (1994) *The Empty Raincoat: Making Sense of the Future*. Hutchinson, London.

Harrison, S., Hunter, D.J. & Pollitt, C. (1992) *Just Managing: Power and Culture in the National Health Service*. Macmillan Press Ltd, Basingstoke.

Hatfield, E., Cacioppo, J.T. & Rapson, R.L. (1994) *Emotional Contagion*. Studies in Emotion and Social Interaction. Cambridge University Press/Editions de la Maison des Sciences de l'Homme, Paris.

Hawthorne, D.L. & Yurkovitch, N.J. (1995) Science, technology, caring and the professions: are they compatible? *Journal of Advanced Nursing*, **21**, 1087–91.

Herd, B., Herd, A. & Mathers, N. (1995) The wizard and the gatekeeper: of castles and contracts. *British Medical Journal*, **310**, 1042–4.

Hickman, C.R. & Silva, M.A. (1984) *Creating Excellence: Managing Corporate Culture Strategy and Change in the New Age*. George Allen & Unwin, London.

Hunsaker, P.L. & Alessandra, A.J. (1980) *The Art of Managing People*. Prentice-Hall, Englewood Cliffs, NJ.

Hutton, W. (1995) A state of decay. *The Guardian.* 18 September.

Illich, I. (1976) *Limits to Medicine: Medical Nemesis: The Expropriation of Health.* Marion Boyars, London.

James, N. (1992) Care, work and carework: a synthesis? In: *Policy Issues in Nursing,* (eds J. Robinson, A. Gray & R. Elkan). Open University Press, Milton Keynes.

Johnson, T., Larkin, J. & Saks, M. (eds) (1995) *Health Professions and the State in Europe.* Routledge, London.

Jones, L.J. (1994) *The Social Context of Health and Health Work.* Macmillan Press Ltd, Basingstoke.

Kasl, S.V. & Cooper, C.L. (eds) (1995) *Research Methods in Stress and Health Psychology.* John Wiley & Sons, Chichester.

Klein, R. (1995) *The New Politics of the NHS.* 3rd edn. Longman, London.

Larkin, G. (1995) State control and the health professions in the United Kingdom. In: *Health Professions and the State in Europe,* (eds T. Johnson, G. Larkin and M Saks). Routledge, London.

Leddy, S. & Pepper, J.M. (1992) *Conceptual Bases of Professional Nursing.* J.B. Lippincott Company, Philadelphia, PA.

Lewis, J. (1992) Providers, 'consumers', the state and the delivery of health-care services in twentieth century Britain. In: *Medicine in Society: Historical Essays,* (ed. A Wear). Cambridge University Press, Cambridge.

Lightfoot, J. (1995) Identifying needs and setting priorities: issues of theory, policy and practice. *Health and Social Care in the Community,* **3,** 105–14.

Little, J.M. (1995) *Humane Medicine.* Cambridge University Press, Cambridge.

Lundin, R.W. (1991) *Theories and Systems of Psychology.* 4th edn. D.C. Heath & Company, Lexington, MA.

Mackay, L. (1993) *Conflicts in Care: Medicine and Nursing.* Chapman & Hall, London.

Marelli, T.M. (1993) *The Nurse Manager's Survival Guide – Practical Answers to Everyday Problems.* Mosby, St Louis, MO.

May, A. (1995) Game of patients. *The Guardian,* 1 November.

May, C. (1995) Patient autonomy and the politics of professional relationships. *Journal of Advanced Nursing,* **21,** 83–7.

Morgan, M., Calnan, M. & Manning, N. (1988) *Sociological Approaches to Health and Medicine.* Routledge, London.

Morton-Cooper, A. (1995) *Clinical support* not *supervision.* Paper presented at the National Assessor's Conference, Thames Valley University, 22 June.

Morton-Cooper, A. & Palmer, A. (1993) *Mentoring & Preceptorship: A Guide to Support Roles in Clinical Practice.* Blackwell Science, Oxford.

Newell, S. (1995) *The Healthy Organization – Fairness, Ethics and Effective Management.* Routledge, London.

Newton, T., Handy, J. & Fineman, S. (1995) *'Managing' Stress: Emotions and Power at Work.* Sage, London.

Nichols, K.A. (1984) *Psychological Care in Physical Illness.* Chapman & Hall, London.

Nolan, M. & Grant, G. (1993) Service evaluation: time to open both eyes. *Journal of Advanced Nursing*, **18**, 1434–42.

Oakley, A. (1993) *Essays on Women, Medicine & Health*. Edinburgh University Press, Edinburgh.

Oliver, M. (1992) Doubts about preventing coronary heart disease. *British Medical Journal*, **304**, 393–4.

Park, K. (1992) Medicine and society in medieval Europe. In: *Medicine in Society: Historical Essays*, (ed. A. Wear). Cambridge University Press, Cambridge.

Parkinson, B. (1995) *Ideas and Realities of Emotion*. Routledge, London.

Parkinson, B. & Colman, A.M. (1995) *Emotion and Motivation*. Longman, London.

Perkins, H. (1989) *The Rise of Professional Society: England Since 1880*. Routledge, London.

Peters, T.J. & Waterman, R.H. (1982) *In Search of Excellence: Lessons from America's Best-run Companies*. Harper and Row, New York.

Pettigrew, A., Ferlie, E. & McKee, L. (1992) *Shaping Strategic Change – Making Change in Large Organizations: the Case of the National Health Service*. Sage, London.

Radical Statistics Health Group (1995) NHS 'indicators of success': what do they tell us? *British Medical Journal*, **310**, 1045–50.

Radley, A. (1994) *Making Sense of Illness: the Social Psychology of Health & Disease*. Sage, London.

Rafaeli, A. & Sutton, R.I. (1995) Expression of emotion as part of the work role. In: *Psychological Dimensions of Organizational Behaviour*, (ed. B.M. Staw), 2nd edn, pp. 114–128. Prentice-Hall, Englewood Cliffs, NJ.

Renade, W. (1994) *A future for the NHS: Health Care in the 1990s*. Longman, London.

Research Unit in Health and Behavioural Change (1993) *Changing the Public Health*. John Wiley & Sons/University of Edinburgh, Chichester.

Russell, D. (1995) *Women, Madness & Medicine*. Polity Press in association with Blackwell Publishers, Cambridge.

Salvage, J. (1992) The new nursing: empowering patients or empowering nurses? In: *Policy Issues in Nursing* (eds J. Robinson, A. Gray & R. Elkan). Open University Press, Milton Keynes.

Samson, C. (1995) Madness and psychiatry. In: *Medical Power and Medical Sociology*, 2nd edn (ed. B.S. Turner). Sage, London.

Schubert-Lehnhardt, V. (1995) Who should be responsible for a nation's health? In: *Reforming Health Care: The Philosophy and Practice of International Health Reform*, (ed. D. Seedhouse), pp. 167–170. John Wiley & Sons, Chichester.

Seedhouse, D. (1988) *Ethics: the Heart of Health Care*. John Wiley & Sons, Chichester.

Seedhouse, D. (ed.) (1995) *Reforming Health Care: The Philosophy and Practice of International Health Reform*. John Wiley & Sons, Chichester.

Spitzer, R.L. & Williams, J. (eds) (1987) *Diagnostic and Statistical Manual of Mental Disorders*. American Psychiatric Association, Washington, DC.

Strike, A.J. (1995) *Human Resources in Health Care – A Manager's Guide.* Blackwell Science, Oxford.

Thompson, G. (ed.) (1994) *The United States in the Twentieth Century: Markets.* The Open University/Hodder & Stoughton Publishing, Milton Keynes.

Thorne, S. (1993) Health belief systems in perspective. *Journal of Advanced Nursing,* **18**, 1931–41.

Timmins, N. (1995) *The Five Giants: a Biography of the Welfare State.* Harper-Collins, London.

Toffler, A. (1977) *Future Shock.* Pan Books, London.

Turner, B.S. (1995) *Medical Power and Social Knowledge,* 2nd edn. Sage, London.

Walby, S. Greenwell, J., Mackay, L. & Soothill, K. (1994) *Medicine and Nursing: Professions in a Changing Health Service.* Sage, London.

Wall, A. (1989) *Ethics and the Health Services Manager.* King Edward's Hospital Fund for London, London.

Wall, A. (1995) A manager's view. In: *Ethics – the Patient's Charter,* (ed. V. Tschudin). Scutari Press, London.

Warr, P. (1987) *Work, Unemployment and Mental Health.* Oxford Science Publications, Oxford.

Watson, T.J. (1994) *In Search of Management: Culture, Chaos and Control in Managerial Work.* Routledge, London.

Weatherall, D. (1995) *Science and the Quiet Art: Medical Research and Patient Care.* Oxford University Press, Oxford.

Wedding, D. (ed.) (1995) *Behavior and Medicine,* 2nd edn. Mosby, St. Louis, MO.

WHO (1981) *Health Services in Europe,* Vol. 1. World Health Organization, Copenhagen.

Wilkinson, M.J. (1995) Love is not a marketable commodity: new public management in the British National Health Service. *Journal of Advanced Nursing,* **21**, 980–87.

Witz, A. (1992) *Professions and Patriarchy.* Routledge, London.

Witz, A. (1994) The challenge of nursing. In: *Challenging Medicine,* (eds J. Gabe, D. Kelleher & G. Williams). Routledge, London.

Yukl, G. (1994) *Leadership in Organizations,* 3rd edn. Prentice-Hall, Englewood Cliffs, NJ.

Zola, I.K. (1972) Medicine as an institution of social control. *The Sociological Review,* **20**, 487–503.

Suggested further reading

Carnall, C.A. (1995) *Managing Change in Organizations,* 2nd edn. Prentice-Hall, London.
This is a helpful and authoritative introduction to change management written by a professor of management studies at Henley Management College. Its primary readership is stated to be MBA students, but the book is easily accessible to undergraduate and diploma students.

Hayward, T. (1995) *Ecological Thought – an Introduction.* Polity Press, Cambridge.
This text is an insightful and rewarding read for those who are keen to see political and economic thought rooted in an ecological paradigm. The author's analysis of the 'paradigm of production' is particularly relevant to the debate over rationing of health resources.

Higgs, J. & Jones, M. (eds) (1995) *Clinical Reasoning in the Health Professions.* Butterworth-Heinemann, Oxford.
This book traces the development of clinical reasoning for practitioners of a number of disciplines (notably medicine, physiotherapy, occupational and speech therapy and nursing), and includes a very constructive overview of the use of alternative methods and educational technologies in teaching, clinical reasoning and encouraging what are described as 'clinical reasoning behaviours'.

Sainsbury, R.M. (1988) *Paradoxes.* Cambridge University Press, Cambridge.
I would recommend this book to the 'logically' minded. It is the work of an eminent philosopher and academic who has used paradox to attempt to solve philosophical problems. It contains references from the classic literature on paradoxes for the real enthusiast!

Salaman, G. (1995) *Managing.* Open University Press, Buckingham.
This is a useful introductory text for beginning managers and those requiring an up to date overview. A handy size for those train journeys which always take longer than planned!

Index